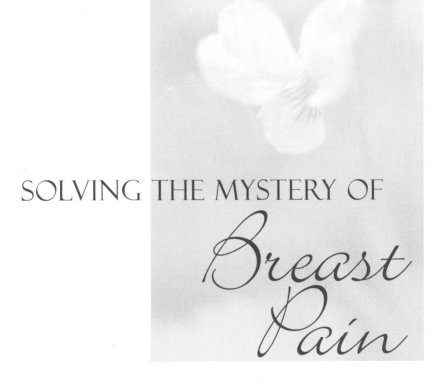

SOLVING THE MYSTERY OF

Breast Pain

JUDY C. KNEECE, RN, OCN
BREAST HEALTH SPECIALIST

Fully Revised Second Edition: 2003; First Edition: 1996
ISBN 1-886665-06-0
Library of Congress Card Number: 96-083810
Printed in the United States of America
Published by EduCare Inc.

To order additional copies of this book, contact:

EduCare Publishing
211 Medical Circle
West Columbia, SC 29169
Phone: 803-796-6100
Fax: 803-796-4150
Internet: www.educareinc.com

Publisher's Cataloging In Publication

Kneece, Judy C.
    Solving the Mystery of Breast Pain
  Judy C. Kneece
    p. cm.
Includes bibliographical references and index
    ISBN: 1-886665-06-0

  1. Breast--Examination. 2. Breast--Diseases. 3. Breast--Cancer. I. Title.

TABLE OF CONTENTS

Chapter 3 *Noncyclic Pain*   31

ACKNOWLEDGMENTS

Henry Patrick Leis, Jr., M.D.
Breast Surgeon, Retired

John Coscia, M.D.
Radiologist, Executive Director
The Comprehensive Breast Center
Don and Sybil Harrington Cancer Center, Amarillo, Texas

Brian Gelfand, M.D., F.A.C.S.
Dedicated Breast Surgeon
Elliot Hospital Breast Center
Manchester, New Hampshire

Kamilia Kozlowski, M.D.
Clinical Diagnostic Breast Radiologist
Knoxville Breast Center, Knoxville, Tennessee

Davis Hook, R.Ph.
Hawthorne Pharmacy, Columbia, South Carolina

**University of South Carolina School of Pharmacy
Drug Information Center**

Debra Strange
Illustrations

Rick Smoak
Photography

About The Author

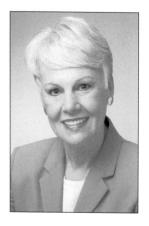

Judy C. Kneece, RN, OCN, is a certified oncology nurse with a specialty in breast cancer and is a MammaCare® Specialist, as well as an author, trainer, and consultant. She presently serves as a national Breast Health Consultant for hospitals and breast centers on the educational and psychosocial needs of the breast patient. She conducts strategic planning and oversees implementation of a comprehensive program of education and support for patients, and trains nurses in a forty-hour training course to fill the role of breast health educator.

Her background as a Breast Health Specialist has allowed her to train thousands of women in breast self-exam skills. It was through this experience that she recognized that women need information about normal and abnormal changes in their breasts and how they can work as a partner with their healthcare providers in monitoring their breast health between clinical exams. She also recognized the need for information by women who have found something suspicious in their breasts, are waiting for an evaluation, or who have high anxiety over monitoring their breasts. To fill this need, she has written this book.

Judy is the author of five books, 35 national journal articles, 291 Patient Education Teaching Topics, *The Breast Health Specialists Manual* and *The Breast Center Strategic Planning Guide*. Her books, *Your Breast Cancer Treatment Handbook*, *Helping Your Mate Face Breast Cancer* and *Finding a Lump In Your Breast*, have all received outstanding reviews in the Journal of the National Cancer Institute. She is also the author of *Solving the Mystery of Breast Pain* and *Solving the Mystery of Breast Discharge*. She is a contributing editor to major women's magazine articles about breast health, including *Redbook*, *Marie Claire*, *Self*, *Good Housekeeping*, *Women's Day* and others.

EduCare's Internet site (www.educareinc.com) launched in 1995, was one of the first breast health sites on the web and presently serves approximately 200,000 people per month.

Judy has led efforts in the past several years to research the topics of recurrent breast cancer and its psychological and social impact, and most recently, sexuality issues after chemotherapy. To gather the information, focus groups of survivors were convened across the nation. Data from these focus groups was collected utilizing interactive computers. The final studies have detailed the experience of these survivors and identified their needs for education and support.

As an instructor, Judy has trained and certified over 1,000 nurses internationally in a forty-hour training course on how to implement programs of education and support for breast health patients in breast centers. In the last ten years she has led an international effort to change the care-delivery of breast cancer patients by (1) identifying breast cancer patient's needs through focus groups, interviews and surveys; (2) instructing nurses on how to deliver patient-focused care in a forty-hour breast health specialist certification program; and (3) leading strategic planning workshops for hospitals to teach how to implement a comprehensive breast care program that includes the psychosocial needs of women.

Judy served as a member of the National Consortium of Breast Centers board of directors for eight years and as the editor of its newsletter, the *Breast Center Bulletin*. She recently served as a guest expert for the American Cancer Society's planning and taping of a new recurrent video series. She presently serves as a member of the Department of Defense Breast Health Scientific Advisory Board representing the interests of breast health patients in the area of educational and psychosocial needs.

As a regular conference speaker and trainer, Judy is best known for her advocacy of the breast cancer patient's psychological and social needs.

DEDICATION

This book is dedicated to **Dr. Henry Patrick Leis, Jr.**, who served as one of my first mentors in the area of breast disease. It was through his gracious sharing of his clinical expertise that I gained much insight into the problems of breast pain and discharge.

As a young physician, Dr. Leis took a fellowship in breast surgery following World War II and spent the remainder of his distinguished career as a dedicated breast surgeon. As a Professor Emeritus of Surgery, Emeritus Chief of the Breast Service and Emeritus Co-Director of the Institute of Breast Diseases at New York Medical College in Valhalla, New York, Dr. Leis made contributions to breast care that still stand as hallmarks of excellence.

His vision of care extended beyond the surgical removal of breast tumors to improving the quality of life for patients. He was the first physician to write instructions and exercises distributed by the American Cancer Society to women on the postsurgical care of their arms. He worked closely with Terese Lasser, the founder of the Reach To Recovery program, to make physical and psychosocial support available to patients. As a result of his work, thousands of women have enjoyed increased degrees of physical and psychological survivorship after breast cancer.

He is the author of numerous surgical textbooks and articles on breast cancer, but his outstanding accomplishment is his personal campaign to promote a multi-disciplinary approach to breast disease. His patient-centered philosophy makes him one of the leading heroes in changing the way breast care is delivered today. His influence will continue to affect women internationally as he has affected me as an educator and a woman.

INTRODUCTION

"At the present, most physicians are ill-trained for the treatment of mastalgia. 90 percent of patients with cyclic pain and 64 percent with noncyclic pain can obtain relief with proper assessment and a combination of nonprescription and prescription drugs."

Dr. Suzanne Klimberg, M.D.
The Breast, 1998

Breast pain is the most common of all breast problems. It would be natural to assume as women that the research in this area is well-documented with clear definitions and guidelines for physicians and other healthcare providers, yet until recently this was not the case. What was written was both poor in quality and clarity. Clinicians had few guidelines and patients were most often offered reassurance after a clinical exam or mammogram that it was not caused by cancer.

Dr. Leis was a pioneer in recognizing and lecturing to physicians about breast pain. He carefully documented patients' complaints, comparing them to future disease, causes, and promoters of different types of pain. It was through his sharing of this information, collected over fifty years of practice, that I have had the privilege to continue to carry the message of understanding the meaning of breast pain to women and nurses—a subject that affects them equally. My goal is to make this common problem understandable and offer observations for management and treatment.

Good breast health to you!

Judy

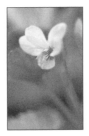

CHAPTER 1

BREAST PAIN

(Breast Mastalgia or Mastodynia)

"My breasts hurt!" "Why are they so painful?" "What can I do about the pain?" "I'm scared! . . . Could this possibly mean I have breast cancer?" You may be experiencing some of the same fears and asking the same questions about your breasts if you have pain. Pain is the most common complaint women have about their breasts. It is also the most feared of any breast change because most women associate pain with cancer.

Breast pain is often the most difficult breast problem to diagnose because it has a vast variety of causes that often require intensive investigation to determine the precipitating factor. Determining the cause of breast pain can require more time to pinpoint than most breast diseases because it often eludes traditional screening evaluations such as clinical exams, mammography exams, and ultrasounds. Breast pain often requires an intensive look into many problems outside of the breast as the cause. Because of the difficulty determining the cause, many women live with breast pain after being told that there were no abnormalities in their screening exams.

The purpose of this book is to help you understand breast pain, its identified causes, and along with your healthcare provider's screening evaluation, help you solve the mystery of what is causing your pain and what you can do about it.

Pain in one or both breasts can cause you much anxiety. The pain may be uncomfortable and annoying, but for the majority of women it is usually not unbearable. What seems unbearable is the fear that it might be cancer. For this reason, you need to work as a partner with your healthcare provider in finding the cause. Studies show that only a very small percentage of breast pain is associated with breast cancer. Almost all breast pain is due to other causes. In fact, pain with breast cancer is uncommon. Less than 10 percent of diagnosed breast cancer patients have any type of pain or discomfort as a symptom. If your healthcare provider doesn't appear overly alarmed when you report you have breast pain, know that it is because most breast pain is usually caused by problems that are not life threatening. However, this does not mean the cause of your pain should not be identified. During the process of identifying the reason for your breast pain, just remember that cancer is usually not the cause.

What Should I Do If I Have Breast Pain?

Breast pain in both breasts, occurring before a menstrual period that is noticeable but not severe is normal for premenopausal women. So the question is, what pain do you need to report to a healthcare provider for evaluation?

Report to a healthcare provider:

- Pain that is persistent (lasting longer than several weeks)
- Pain that is sudden and severe
- Pain along with redness and warmth of breast tissues
- Pain along with a lump in the same breast
- Pain along with discharge from one breast
- Pain in one breast that also has a change in texture of the skin
- Pain that has a large amount of discharge from both breasts, not associated with pregnancy or nursing

Remember:

- Note: Very commonly, bilateral breast pain is an early warning symptom of pregnancy. If your pain began recently and it is possible that you may be pregnant, a pregnancy test is your first step in evaluation.

A healthcare provider's clinical evaluation will include a careful history, a thorough breast exam, a mammogram or an ultrasound if indicated, and possibly a biopsy or culture if an abnormality is found. This examination helps rule out breast cancer as the cause of your pain and in the process often identifies the cause of your pain. Many benign diseases have pain as a symptom and are discussed in this book. For some women the search for the cause of their pain may be difficult and require more than one exam to investigate all the possible causes. During this search your healthcare provider will offer interventions and a plan for pain management.

The first step in determining the cause of your breast pain is having your healthcare provider rule out disease. This book will help you work in partnership with your healthcare provider, to understand the different causes of breast pain, and to find the possible cause of your pain. After ruling out disease, the next step is to determine if your pain is cyclic (regular intervals) or noncyclic (does not occur in cycles). Because these two types of pain are completely different in origin, each type of pain is discussed separately.

Remember:

- Breast pain is most often related to noncancerous causes.
- Breast pain is often difficult to diagnose because of its many causes.
- The first step is to have a healthcare provider rule out any disease in the breasts.

On the next page is a full diagram of the female breast. As you will see the breast is a very complex glandular organ that sits on the chest wall over the pectoralis muscles and ribs. It is an organ that changes daily because of the influence of hormones.

Becoming familiar with your own breast and its function will help you work as a partner with your healthcare provider.

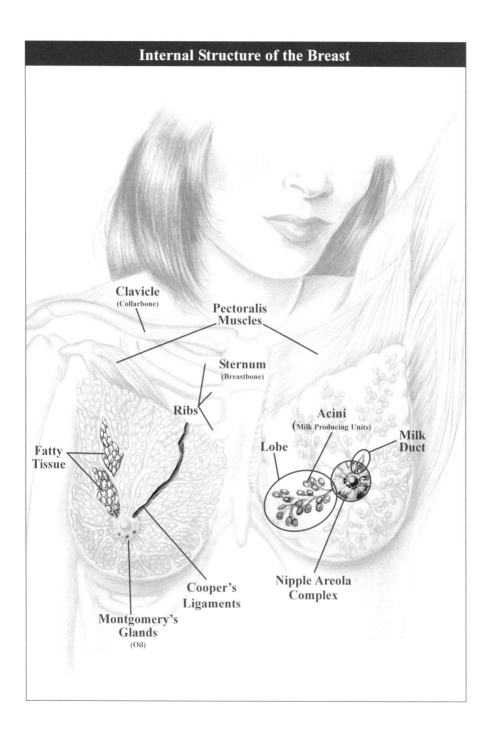

Clavicle
(Collarbone)

Pectoralis
Muscles

Sternum
(Breastbone)

Ribs

Acini
(Milk Producing Units)

Lobe

Milk
Duct

Fatty
Tissue

Cooper's
Ligaments

Nipple Areola
Complex

Montgomery's
Glands
(Oil)

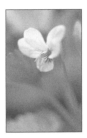

CHAPTER 2

CYCLIC PAIN

The most common pain is cyclic pain. It is called cyclic because the pain corresponds with monthly recurring changes in the levels of your female hormones: estrogen, progesterone and prolactin. These hormone levels rise and fall during your monthly cycle.

We are all familiar with the impact hormone levels have on a woman's ability to become pregnant. At midcycle, an egg is released during ovulation; if the egg is not fertilized, pregnancy does not occur, and the menstrual cycle begins.

We are less familiar with the fact that these fluctuations in hormone levels also cause the breasts to prepare for pregnancy each month—the cells in the ducts of the breasts increase in number, and milk-producing cells (acini) proliferate and produce fluid that is stored in the milk ducts. Right before your menstrual period, approximately 15 to 30 cc (three to six teaspoons) of fluid is stored in each breast. This causes enlargement of your breasts that can create tenderness and pain. Some women are very sensitive to these hormonal changes and about the time of ovulation begin to experience increasing tenderness and breast pain that continues until menstruation occurs. By the end of the menstrual cycle the cyclic pain diminishes.

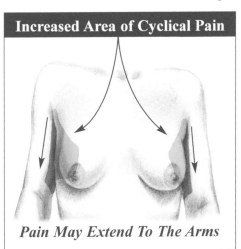

Increased Area of Cyclical Pain

Pain May Extend To The Arms

The clinical description of cyclic breast pain includes:

- Pain that begins at ovulation
- Pain that occurs in both breasts
- Pain that increases until menstruation
- Pain that is significantly relieved during menstruation
- Pain that may be greater in one breast than the other
- Pain that is usually greatest in the upper, outer breast quadrant (from the nipple back toward the armpit)
- Pain that is described as dull and aching, as if the breasts are filled with milk
- Pain that may radiate to the underarm area (axilla) and down the arm to the elbow
- Pain that is experienced by premenopausal women
- Pain that increases several years before the onset of menopause in some women because levels of estrogen become sporadic, rising to very high levels some months
- Pain that is relieved at menopause unless estrogen replacement therapy is being taken (if pain continues after several months contact your healthcare provider to reduce dosage of medication to reduce pain)

How Common is Cyclic Breast Pain?

A study reported in the *Journal of Obstetrics and Gynecology*, "Presence and Impact of Cyclical Mastalgia" (1997), gave an overview of cyclical breast pain in 1,171 women attending a GYN clinic. When the women were interviewed about monthly breast pain, the study revealed the following about their pain and its impact on their lifestyle:

- 69 percent had regular monthly discomfort
- 36 percent had consulted their healthcare provider about their pain
- 11 percent rated their monthly pain as moderate to severe
- 48 percent said it interfered with sexual activity
- 37 percent said it interfered with physical activities performed

- 12 percent said it interfered with social activities
- 8 percent said it interfered with work activities

Other studies have shown the percentage of cyclic pain reported by women interviewed to be as high as 85 percent. The simple fact is that cyclic breast pain is common. Most women experience some change in their breasts during the menstrual cycle, with a small percentage reporting severe pain.

How To Determine If Your Pain Is Cyclic

The best way to determine if your pain is cyclic is to keep a calendar for recording the intensity of your pain each day and to mark the time in your cycle. If your pain is from hormonal changes, you will notice that it begins to increase around ovulation and reaches its peak at the onset of menstruation. It may take one to two months of recording this information to determine if your pain coincides with a change in your hormones. For directions on keeping a monthly record, refer to the pain assessment worksheets and calendars at the back of this book.

Understanding the Role of Reproductive Hormones

A woman's hormones play a large part in her reproductive cycle. The levels vary almost daily. These hormonal changes affect the breast and the uterus. Most women are more aware of hormonal changes because of their menstrual cycle and the potential for pregnancy. However, while the uterus is undergoing changes the breast is also busy preparing for pregnancy. *(See chart on page 21.)*

Hormonal Changes in Menstrual Cycle

Changing levels of hormones cause a woman's body to prepare her uterus for pregnancy. Most menstrual periods have a 28-day cycle, with the beginning of the menstrual flow usually considered day one. During the menstrual flow and for several days after, the hormones estrogen and progesterone are low. At the same time the follicle-stimulating hormone (FHS) and luteinizing hormone (LH) are higher, sending a message to the ovaries to develop an egg (oocyte).

Uterine Changes: (See chart on next page)

Day 1 Menstrual flow begins.

Day 6 One oocyte (sac containing egg) is ready. This oocyte starts making estrogen, which rebuilds the lining of the uterus.

Day 12 LH and FSH cause the follicle (the corpus luteum, a sac in which egg matures) to rupture.

Day 14 The egg is released (ovulation) and the corpus luteum now makes high levels of progesterone to maintain the uterine lining. The egg travels down the tubes as it waits to be fertilized.

Day 28 If the egg is not fertilized the corpus luteum degenerates and the levels of estrogen and progesterone drop greatly. This causes the lining of the uterus to shed and the menstrual bleeding to begin.

Breast Changes: (See chart on next page)

■ Each month the breasts prepare for pregnancy, just like the uterus. They follow a similar path from hormonal stimulation.

■ As estrogen levels rise the first two weeks of the new cycle, the cells in the breast proliferate (increase in number). This part of the cycle is called the proliferative phase of the breast.

■ Ovulation takes place at mid-cycle and the corpus luteum (sac that held the egg) produces progesterone.

■ Increased progesterone levels cause stimulation of the fluid-producing units (acini), and they begin to produce and store fluid (3 to 6 teaspoons) in each breast. This part of the cycle is called the secretory phase.

■ During the two weeks (secretory phase) before a period, the breasts begin to feel fuller day by day. The week before menstruation begins, the breasts often feel heavy, as if they are full of milk. During this time many women experience breast pain. This pain ranges from a mild feeling of discomfort to very painful.

Just as some women experience menstrual cramps, some women experience breast pain. The difference is that breast pain precedes menstrual cramps. Both are related to the normal hormonal changes of the body. Neither are a sign of disease.

Reproductive Hormones Impact on the Breast

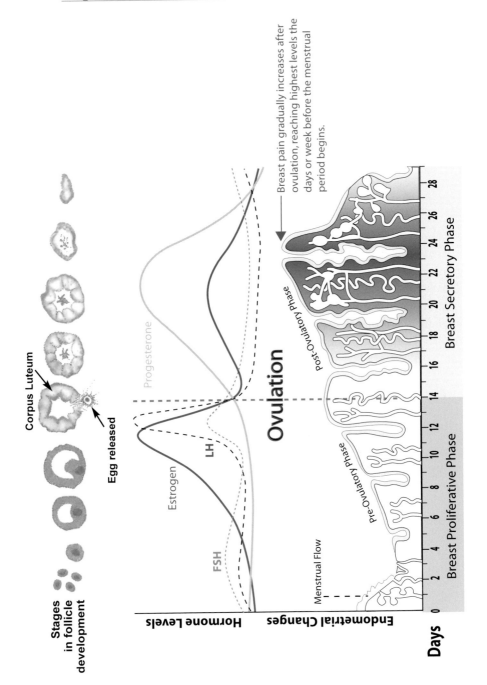

Factors Contributing to Cyclic Pain

After you have explored with your healthcare provider the cause of your pain and found that it is cyclic and not related to a treatable disease, there are specific remedies you can try. Once discovering that their pain is cyclic, many women find that their pain is still annoying but no longer quite as worrisome. However, it is helpful to know that there are known contributing factors that can increase the discomfort of cyclic pain, and that there are simple remedies that may reduce it. Factors that may increase cyclic pain include the consumption of caffeine products, high sodium diets, and high fat diets.

Caffeine

Caffeine is a methylxanthine, a chemical that some women find significantly increases their symptoms of fibrocystic changes (such as increased lumpiness, tenderness, or breast cysts) as well as their pain. Some studies have shown caffeine to be an influencing factor and others have not. What matters is how you respond to caffeine. Caffeine reduction or elimination is something you can try and will not cost you anything. Some women report that the reduction or elimination of caffeine is helpful; others report that it has no effect. Only a trial of eliminating caffeine from your diet can help determine if caffeine contributes to your pain.

When we talk about caffeine, most people first think of coffee. However, caffeine is found not only in coffee, but also in tea, soft drinks, chocolate, and many over-the-counter medications and herbal products. Reducing the amount of caffeine and caffeine-containing products in your diet may reduce cyclic pain. This is a simple change you can make in your diet. But remember, it may take months to determine the effect caffeine has on your body. One or two weeks of reduced caffeine is not an adequate trial for understanding caffeine's effects on breast pain. Refer to Chapter 4 for a caffeine reduction plan and a list of common caffeine-containing products.

High Sodium Diets

Large amounts of sodium (salt) in one's diet may also increase cyclic breast pain because a high sodium diet causes your body to retain more fluid. The increase in breast fluid from normal hormonal changes is compounded by a high sodium diet, and your pain may also be increased. Reducing salt in the diet, especially during the second half of the menstrual cycle, reduces fluid retention and thus may reduce breast pain for some.

Reducing the salt in your diet is also an intervention you can try that will not cost anything and allows you to determine for yourself if it is helpful. For general health reasons, we know that a diet lower in sodium-saturated products is healthier. You can easily reduce the sodium in your diet by eating more fresh fruits and vegetables while eating fewer salty snack foods and commercially prepared foods. Drinking more water also helps the body to eliminate excessive sodium. Sodium is removed from the body through the kidneys. Therefore, adequate amounts of fluid are necessary for this removal. Drinking large amounts of water (eight glasses a day) is helpful. If you do not like water, try adding a bit of fresh lemon to cold water to alter the taste. Water is better that many soft drinks and beers that are very high in sodium.

Monitor your intake of sodium. The recommended daily allowance of sodium is from 2,000 to 3,000 milligrams a day. Many women are surprised to learn that they consume much more than the recommended allowance of sodium. But remember, sodium is necessary for good health. Your goal is not a severely restricted sodium diet, but rather a diet that involves moderate salt consumption.

To monitor and reduce your sodium intake:

- Read all labels on food and drinks for sodium content
- Avoid using the salt shaker or adding extra salt to food
- Replace salt with lemon, herbs, and salt substitutes
- Substitute fresh vegetables and soups for canned varieties
- Avoid processed and marinated meats
- Monitor your use of ketchup, mustard, salad dressings, pickles, bacon bits, soy sauce and other condiments
- Substitute water for soft drinks or beer
- Substitute fresh fruit for salty snack foods

High Fat Diets

The amount of dietary fat in your diet can influence your hormonal levels. High fat diets increase the production of estrogen in the body, and low fat diets can reduce the amount of estrogen your body makes. Reducing the fat in your diet can reduce the amount of stimulation your breasts receive from your own hormones and may help reduce your breast pain. It is recommended that only 20 to 25 percent of your diet come from fat. Some physicians recommend a diet as low as 15 percent in fat for severe breast pain that is cyclic. Find a fat gram book and learn to count your fat grams, keeping your daily total of grams in the recommended range. Increasing your consumption of fresh fruits, vegetables and whole grains is one of the easiest ways because they are naturally low in fat. This is another simple, healthy way to address breast pain causes and possibly find relief.

To monitor and reduce the fat in your diet:

- Read labels for percentage of fat content and fat grams per serving
- Read labels for kinds of fat and avoid animal fat
- Limit the number of fat grams you eat daily
- Eat more chicken, turkey and fish instead of red meat
- Broil or bake meat; use a nonstick skillet and cooking spray
- Buy fat-free or low-fat salad dressings and mayonnaise; use sparingly
- Buy low-fat cheese
- Eat more pasta and cereals
- Drink skim or lowfat milk
- Eat nonfat yogurt
- Cook vegetables with no fat

Types of Cyclic Pain Management

Treatment of cyclic breast pain may consist of dietary supplements, mechanical interventions, and prescription medications.

Dietary Supplements

It is suggested that you consult your healthcare provider before taking any dietary supplements discussed in this chapter for the treatment of your pain.

In the early 1980s, Dr. Henry Leis conducted one of the first studies in which women having cyclical breast pain were treated using dietary interventions. A total of 721 women were placed on a low-fat, high fiber diet supplemented with vitamins A, C, E and selenium. At the end of the study, 81 percent of the women reported a reduction of pain and tenderness and 39 percent had a clinical exam revealing a decrease in nodularity (lumpiness).

Addressing cyclic breast pain with dietary changes and supplements has become one of the first interventions for cyclic breast pain. Today, many women are looking for non-pharmaceutical interventions that come from supplements and diet. One of the most respected leaders in women's health in the area of natural and complementary medicine is Tori Hudson, N.D. The author of the *Women's Encyclopedia of Natural Medicine*, Dr. Hudson recommends that women with benign breast problems including pain:

- Avoid caffeine
- Lower dietary fat to 20 percent
- Increase dietary fiber
- Increase intake of seafood and seaweed

Supplements Recommended:

- Vitamin E (natural)—400 - 800 IU (international units) daily
- Evening Primrose Oil—1,500 mg twice daily
- Beta Carotene—50,000 - 150,000 IU (international units) daily
- Natural progesterone cream ¼ to ½ teaspoon applied to breasts twice a day from ovulation to menstruation

Major supplements used for breast pain:

Vitamin E

Vitamin E has been used for years for the treatment of benign breast disease. Some studies have confirmed its success while others have not proved any benefit. Since vitamin E in dosages of 400 - 800 IU per day is proven completely safe, this is a simple and appropriate treatment to try for breast pain.

Evening Primrose Oil (Oenothera biennis)

Evening Primrose Oil (linolenic acid) is an essential fatty acid occurring in some fish oils and many seed-derived oils. Linolenic acid functions as an anti-inflammatory agent in the breast by stabilizing adenylate cyclase (an enzyme that is activated by certain hormones) and is the only natural therapy to be scientifically studied in relation to breast pain. Studies have shown that Evening Primrose Oil significantly reduces breast pain in approximately 50 percent of women with cyclical breast pain. The dosage used in the studies was three grams a day for three months. This is a naturally occurring essential fatty acid and the only reported side effect was mild nausea by a small percentage of women. Evening Primrose Oil is the 'first line' of treatment for breast pain in European countries. Other omega-6 fatty acids that may have beneficial effects but have not been studied in relationship to benign breast disease are flaxseed oil, black currant oil and borage oil.

Mechanical Interventions for Cyclic Pain

A variety of mechanical interventions may help reduce cyclic breast pain. These include bras, hot or cold applications, and breast massages. Because some of the pain in the breasts is due to their size increasing when fluid fills and stretches the tissues, interventions that prevent movement or remove some of the fluid may reduce pain. These methods are all free or inexpensive and have no negative side effects. They work by reducing the stretching and irritation of nerve fibers. Keep your healthcare provider informed as you explore ways to reduce your pain.

Bras

A properly fitted bra that minimizes movement of the breasts is effective for many women. Wearing a sports bra when sleeping and when exercising is also suggested for women experiencing breast pain. Avoid going braless as this allows the breast fibers to stretch; free movement increases pain. A well-fitted bra stabilizes the breasts on the chest wall and prevents stretching of the nerve fibers. In one study, 75 percent of women reported pain reduction by wearing a well-fitted bra and sleeping in a bra. Large-breasted women have found that special bras with wide straps may also reduce pain. If you have a reddened area from a bra strap pressing into your shoulder when you remove your bra, this is a sign that your bra does not fit properly and that you need a wider bra strap. If you cannot find one in a department store, check at your local prosthesis store. They carry wide-strap bras and are experts in bra fitting. For any woman experiencing breast pain, a properly fitted bra is an important first step to pain management.

Hot or Cold Applications

During acute episodes of breast pain before your menstrual cycle, applying heat or cold may reduce pain. A heating pad, hot bath, or shower is helpful for some women. Others find that an ice pack applied to the painful areas of the breasts eases their pain. Heat or cold may reduce swelling and thus reduce pain. There are no clinical studies on these interventions, only anecdotal reports from women saying, "this seemed to help my pain." Once again, trying either will not cost anything and may be helpful.

Breast Massage

Breast massage can also reduce pain by helping to remove excess fluid through the lymphatic system. Massage therapists have proven this with breast cancer patients who have breast lymphedema after lumpectomy. Massage is an option for reducing cyclical breast pain if it is caused from fluid accumulation in the breast.

Instructions for Self-Massage:

1. Put lotion on your hands to reduce friction.

2. Make dime-size round circles over all of the breast tissues just as you do during breast self-exam. Start at the bra line and make straight lines of small circles up to your collar bone.

3. Repeat another row starting at the bra line until all breast tissue is covered. This increases the removal of fluid from breast tissues.

A breast massage is easily performed in the shower when your hands and breasts are soapy.

Prescription Medications

If you have tried all the previously described interventions (made changes in your diet, tried dietary supplements, etc.) but have found no relief from your pain, your healthcare provider may prescribe medication as a final remedy. Since cyclic breast pain is hormonally stimulated, prescription medications may be used to lower the levels of circulating hormones or to balance them out. Prescription medications frequently used include birth control pills, progesterone, Danazol, and Bromocriptine.

Birth Control Pills

Some women find relief from cyclic pain after taking a low-dose birth control pill prescribed by their healthcare provider. The pill suppresses ovarian production of hormones and replaces it with an average synthetic dose of both estrogen and progesterone. If the replacement pill dosage is lower than the natural body's hormones, pain is relieved. However it is possible that the levels in the pill may be higher and the pain may be increased and not relieved. This again is often a trial and error attempt to control pain, but one that has shown to reduce cyclic pain for many women. This intervention has proved extremely helpful for perimenopausal women who experience sporadically high levels of estrogen causing breast pain right before onset of menopause.

Progesterone

Progesterone may be prescribed when a deficiency in progesterone in relationship to estrogen is suspected. Two medical doctors treating hormonal balance in women, Dr. Jesse Handley of the Malibu Health Center and Dr. John R. Lee, retired physician and author, call the condition estrogen dominance. In their book, *What Your Doctor May Not Tell You About Premenopause–Balance Your Hormones and Your Life From Thirty to Fifty*, they offer suggestions about the use of natural progesterone, dietary supplements and diet to treat changes in hormonal function, including breast pain. In their book, they present case studies and their rational for prescribing the various interventions. The estrogen dominance concept and their suggested treatments have been well received by women and some medical professionals because their suggestions are natural, most do not require prescriptions, and women report success with the treatments.

A compounding pharmacist can make natural progesterone into a lozenge, pill, cream or a vaginal suppository. Progesterone crème, applied directly to the breasts, is being recommended by some physicians after proving effective in France. There are now saliva tests to measure hormonal levels to determine if your estrogen/progesterone is in or out of balance. Your compounding pharmacist can refer you to healthcare providers in your area using natural hormonal therapies and saliva testing. You can locate a compounding pharmacist by looking in the yellow pages of your telephone book or calling their national association number (1-800-927-4227) and giving them your zip code to locate a pharmacy near you. They can provide you with names of healthcare providers who prescribe natural progesterone replacement.

Danazol

Danazol (a male hormone) is an approved prescription drug by the Food and Drug Administration for the treatment of breast pain. It eliminates most normal hormonal fluctuations in the female because it is a male hormone. Therefore, side effects, including unwanted hair growth, weight gain, menstrual irregularities, headaches, nausea and depression may be experienced with the medication. It is also expensive; it can cost approximately $200 a month. Danazol is usually only prescribed for severe cases of breast pain after less aggressive treatments have proven unsuccessful.

Tamoxifen

Tamoxifen, an anti-estrogen (with some estrogen like effects), is being used in prevention trials for breast cancer. It has been found to be effective for breast pain, but its use has to be balanced against increased risk for endometrial cancer. This drug is also given to breast cancer patients to reduce recurrence of breast cancer. Tamoxifen may be an option for women who qualify for high-risk breast cancer prevention studies after evaluation by a physician specializing in high-risk breast cancer. It is not recommended for the general population at this time.

Bromocriptine

Bromocriptine is a non-hormonal drug that blocks the production of prolactin (a hormone that promotes breast milk production), and may reduce breast pain. Potential side effects are nausea, headaches, dizziness, and constipation. The drug can be given vaginally by suppository to reduce nausea.

Medication Effectiveness

It usually takes two months to evaluate the effectiveness of medications. Since most medications have some side effects, it is best to try less aggressive methods before resorting to prescription medications. In chapter 3 we will discuss other prescription medications that are used to treat conditions of hypothyroid and galactorrhea that also are associated with breast pain.

Remember:

- Cyclic breast pain is related to the monthly changes in the female hormones
- Most women have some degree of monthly cyclic discomfort
- Cyclic pain has no relationship to cancer
- Cyclic pain can be determined by keeping a monthly record of levels of pain in relationship to menstrual cycle
- Diet and dietary supplements may help some women
- Wearing a well-fitted bra may help to reduce pain
- Severe cyclic pain can be treated with prescription medications

---

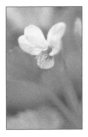

CHAPTER 3

NONCYCLIC PAIN

Noncyclic pain differs from cyclic pain in that it has no relationship to the changing hormonal levels of the menstrual cycle. Noncyclic pain has been linked to benign breast disease, musculoskeletal (muscles/bones) injury or disease, breast or chest area injury, and least often, cancer.

Noncyclic pain has the following characteristics:

- May be continuous, or it may only occur from time to time
- Usually localized to a specific area in one breast, commonly called "target zone pain" or "trigger point pain," indicating that the pain is localized in one area or can be replicated by movement or pressure
- Described as a sharp, stabbing or burning sensation

Benign Breast Diseases

Benign breast diseases are conditions in the breast that may cause problems such as pain, an abnormality on a mammogram, or changes found during a self or clinical breast exam. These conditions are not cancerous and are not life-threatening.

Benign breast disease/conditions that may cause noncyclic pain:

- Cysts—fluid filled sacs
- Fibroadenoma—tumor of fibrous tissues
- Galactocele—fluid filled sac of breast milk
- Mastitis—infection of breast ducts
- Breast abscess—collection of pus in one area

- Duct ectasia—inflammation or infection in and around milk ducts
- Cellulitis—inflammation of the tissues of the breast
- Mondor's disease—inflammation of a breast vein
- Shingles—viral infection caused by herpes zoster (chickenpox virus)
- Hematoma—bruising with collection of blood in one area caused by a direct blow to the breast

All these conditions are benign changes in the breast that need identification, and some require treatment by a healthcare provider. They may or may not have pain as a symptom. A healthcare provider can usually identify these noncancerous diseases during a physical exam with or without a mammogram or ultrasound; occasionally a culture or biopsy is necessary. If your breast pain is ever accompanied by fever, redness of the skin, or warmth in the breast, seek immediate attention from a healthcare provider.

Cysts, fibroadenomas, and galactoceles are less likely to cause pain than the other conditions. Signs and symptoms of other benign diseases causing pain vary, as does the treatment for the condition. What they all have in common besides pain is that they are benign, and not cancerous.

Mastitis

Lactational mastitis is an inflammation that is most often seen in women who are breastfeeding. However, mastitis may occur at any time. Bacteria enter the breasts, usually through the nipple, and invade the ducts. The bacteria cause localized areas of inflammation and infection, producing redness starting in one quadrant that is accompanied by pain that increases gradually. The breast becomes swollen, tender and warm. Infection can quickly spread to other quadrants of the breast. A fever of 101° F degrees or more and flu-like symptoms are common. The pain can become severe in a short period of time.

Antibiotics are usually very effective in treating the infection and should be started as soon as symptoms appear. Symptoms usually improve two to three days after medication is started. Pain is reduced as the antibiotics take effect in reducing the infection. The entire course of antibiotics prescribed by the healthcare provider should be taken. If the redness and pain do not respond to the antibiotics in several days, call your healthcare provider.

Breast Abscess

About 10 percent of mastitis cases will form an abscess—a collection of pus contained in one area of the breast. This area will feel hard, painful and warm to the touch. An abscess has a localized area of pain. Mastitis pain may be more generalized in the breast. Some abscesses will respond to antibiotic treatment if it is started early. However, some do not respond or may be too large, or very painful. These may require that a healthcare provider drain the area surgically. Draining the area of the abscess reduces pain immediately. Because some abscesses tend to recur, some healthcare providers prefer surgical removal.

The most common site for a breast abscess is under the areola in the area of the ducts. Report any pain with tenderness and warmth of the tissues to a healthcare provider immediately so that treatment with antibiotics can be started.

Cellulitis

Cellulitis is an infection of the skin or connective tissues of the breast. It can occur when lymphatic drainage has been reduced by lymph node removal from surgery or radiation therapy. Women who have had lumpectomies have the potential to have cellulitis in the breast anytime after surgery. The same is true for women who have had a mastectomy; the chest wall is subject to infection. This condition is also common in diabetics and immuno-suppressed individuals.

Infection starts in one area of the breast or chest wall, causing it to become tender, swollen, red, painful, and warm to the touch. If left untreated, the infection can spread quickly. Fever and flu-like symptoms may occur. Cellulitis needs immediate treatment with an antibiotic. Pain is reduced gradually after medication is started; symptoms usually improve greatly the first day and are relieved within two to three days. However, all medication should be taken as prescribed. A well-fitted bra will help stabilize the breast and prevent pain caused by movement. Cellulitis can be recurrent and require treatment multiple times. Some infections require IV antibiotics because of their severity.

Mammary Duct Ectasia (Plasma Cell Mastitis or Periductal Mastitis)

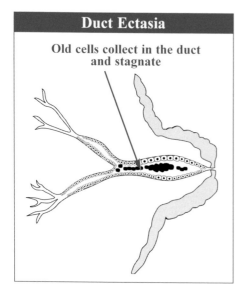

Duct Ectasia

Old cells collect in the duct and stagnate

Normal ducts are line with one or two layers of cells. Mammary duct ectasia is a condition that occurs most frequently in women immediately before and after menopause. It may occur in one, several or all of the ducts on one or both breasts.

Ducts located beneath the nipple become filled and dilated with the cells that line the ducts. This occurs because of stagnation, and not because of a blockage. This accumulated debris appears as a thick, white to greenish-gray to blackish discharge from one, several or all of the nipple openings. The discharge can cause the nipple to itch and become irritated.

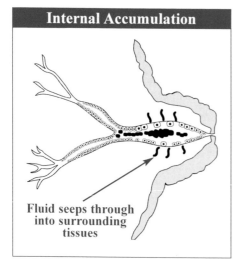

Internal Accumulation

Fluid seeps through into surrounding tissues

The internal accumulation of debris in the duct can also cause a break in the cell walls (called mucosal ulceration) that can cause a bloody discharge. This ulceration causes the tissues around the ducts to swell from a chemical inflammatory reaction to the leaking fluid from inside the ducts. During this inflammatory progression of the condition, pain varies from mild to severe.

Inflammation

Tissues around duct become inflamed, painful and will eventually harden

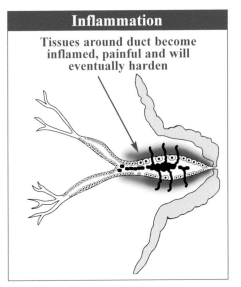

The inflammation causes the tissues around the ducts to become fibrosed (thickened and hardened). During this time pain may be intense. The inflammation can develop into an infection (mastitis) and may even develop into an abscess (a localized collection of pus). Antibiotics will usually resolve the infection, but, occasionally, surgery is required to remove the abscessed duct(s).

Nipple Inversion

Late stage disease often causes nipple inversion

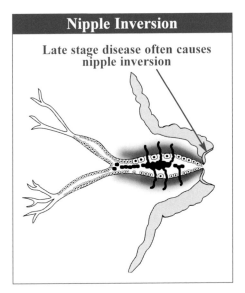

Late stage progression of the disease will often cause nipple inversion. Mammary duct ectasia is not a cancerous condition. Smoking greatly increases the percentage of duct ectasia conditions that develop into chronic infections and abscesses. Duct ectasia can become a chronic problem with periods of remission and then exacerbations.

Mondor's Syndrome

Mondor's syndrome is an inflamed vein in the breast, resulting from a clot. This rare condition may also be called "breast phlebitis" or "superficial periphlebitis." The inflammation of the vein may occur after trauma, muscular strain, radiation therapy, surgical procedures, or occur spontaneously in women with large breasts.

The inflamed vein will be painful and tender along its length. The area may feel like a thick cord in the breast. The pain may last from one to six weeks and can be severe. You may be able to feel the cord-like vein for several months after the pain subsides. The thickened vein may be visible on the surface of the breast. It may also cause skin retraction along the path of the vein. Pain medication may be prescribed; no other treatment is necessary other than wearing a well-fitted bra night and day to stabilize the breast to the chest wall. The condition resolves itself over a period of time.

Shingles (Herpes Zoster)

Herpes zoster of the breast is rare but can occur. The condition is just like shingles on any other part of the body caused by the herpes zoster virus (chicken pox). The outbreak is preceded by pain in the breast that may be severe, and is accompanied with fatigue, and fever. The pain is almost always on one side only (unilateral). Eventually after the pain and fever, small blisters occur on the skin in groups of 8 - 10 and are from 2 - 3 mm (very small) in size. A healthcare provider will prescribe medication for pain and treatment of the virus, along with topical medications to reduce the pain from the blisters. The total duration of the outbreak may be from 10 days to 5 weeks. The condition is more common in people who have weakened immune systems.

Hematoma

Hematoma is a collection of blood under the skin caused by an injury to the area causing internal bleeding. This can happen after a blow to the breast, a breast biopsy, or breast surgery. The area will be painful and a palpable lump can usually be felt in the area of the pain. If the pain is tolerable, a well-fitted bra should be worn day and night to reduce the pain caused by breast movement. If the pain becomes severe, aspiration using a fine needle to withdraw the blood may be necessary to relieve the pain.

Musculoskeletal Conditions Causing Pain

When benign disease is not present and the pain is noncyclic, a common cause is a musculoskeletal (muscle/bones) condition. Musculoskeletal conditions include a pinched nerve, degenerative conditions (such as scoliosis, arthritis, and osteoporosis), and costochondritis.

Pinched Nerve

The most common condition causing noncyclic breast pain is a pinched nerve in the back cervical spine area. If the pain is caused by pressure on a nerve and is referred from the back, usually only one breast will be painful. Another clue as to the discomfort being caused by a pinched nerve is that the arm may also be painful.

To check for this pain, a healthcare provider may ask the patient to elevate her arm (on the painful side) over her head. The healthcare provider, standing behind the patient, lifts the painful breast toward the breastbone and applies pressure in the mid-underarm area. If the pain is coming from a pinched nerve, this will cause a very tender area to radiate pain into the breast.

Degenerative Conditions

Previous occurrences of a back injury, scoliosis, arthritis, or osteoporosis also have the potential to cause pain to the chest area, appearing to be breast pain. If you have a history of any of these degenerative conditions, this may be the cause of your pain. Women who suffer falls in accidents that injure the back may experience breast pain the week(s) following the incident. This pain is referred from the back and is treated by taking care of the underlying cause of the pain.

Costochondritis or Tietze's Syndrome

Another cause of musculoskeletal breast pain is Tietze's syndrome or costochondritis caused by inflammation of the cartilage between the ribs. Tietze's syndrome has swelling at the rib cartilage junction; costochondritis has no noticeable swelling. The pain is from inflammation and neither condition involves infection or an abscess. The pain originates in the area of the breastbone and ribs. It usually occurs on one side of the chest. Because it occurs in

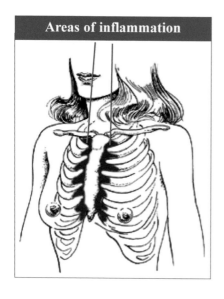

Areas of inflammation

the area of the breast, women often think it is breast pain when it is actually the cartilage under the breast that is the source of pain.

The most common cause of costochondritis is a strain of the rib cage caused by heavy lifting, activities that stretch the upper body, or activities requiring repetitious stretching movement. The condition can also occur from the strain of coughing or weight lifting. Any of the seven costochondral junctions may be affected, and more than one site is affected in 90 percent of cases. The second to fifth costochondral junctions are the most common areas involved.

Women are more likely to have costochondritis than men. In one study of patients diagnosed with costochondritis, 70 percent were women and 30 percent were men. This condition occurs frequently with young mothers from lifting their children. Female athletes suffer more often from costochondritis pain than other women.

Costochondritis pain characteristics:

- Increases with chest movements, deep breaths, or exertion

- Decreases when being still, breathing shallow, or a change of position that relieves pressure on the area

- May feel as a sharp and stabbing pain when acute, or it may be a nagging, dull aching or a pressure-like pain when chronic

- May be localized to one area or pain can radiate extensively over the chest wall if numerous costochondral junctions are involved

- Onset occurs gradually over several hours after activity that stretches the cartilage

- Acute episodes may progress to very severe pain requiring pain medications

Physical exam reveals:

- Pain in the area of the ribs and sternum that increases when pressure is applied to sternum (reproducible pain when pressing on the sternum is the most reliable sign of costochondritis; if the pain is not reproducible, it is not costochondritis)

- Pain increases when moving the rib cage or when taking a deep breath

- Lifting the arms over head severely increases the pain

- During an acute stage, the pain is so intense that it is often mistaken for heart problems, requiring an EKG to rule it out

- During an acute attack, breathing becomes more rapid because of the inability to take a deep breath

Costochondritis pain is identified from its symptoms. Acute pain may require prescription pain medications. Continued treatment consists of non-steroidal anti-inflammatory drugs (NSAIDs) such as ibuprofen to reduce and control the pain. NSAIDs affect the prostaglandins, chemicals in the body that cause inflammation. Because the pain is from inflammation, anti-inflammatory medications usually ease the pain in 24 to 48 hours. While effective, NSAIDS can also cause stomach irritation. Treatments for chronic costochondritis include taking NSAIDs on a regular schedule during the period of inflammation and avoiding the activity that caused the strain on the rib cage. If the pain remains chronic, steroid injections into the rib/sternum junction may be given to reduce inflammation. Costochondritis may recur if the cartilage is reinjured.

Miscellaneous Causes of Noncyclic Breast Pain:

- Infected teeth may cause pain to refer to the breast

- Angina and congestive heart failure may mimic breast pain

- An incisional breast biopsy, lumpectomy, breast reduction or breast augmentation surgery may cause a sharp, shooting pain in the area of the scar for months or even years after surgery

- Breast implants can cause inflammation of the chest wall, causing pain

- Silicone granulomas (a collection of free silicone from a breast implant that has formed into a small lump) may cause an inflammatory reaction in the tissues around it and cause pain

- Breast implant (saline or silicone) contracture (a fibrous shell the body forms around an implant that causes it to change in shape) may cause pain

- Gastrointestinal conditions including hiatal hernia, reflux condition and ulcers may cause discomfort in the chest area and be mistaken for pain originating in the breast

Physiological Conditions Promoting Breast Pain

Physiological conditions that may cause noncyclic breast pain include hypothyroidism, galactorrhea, and cancer.

Hypothyroidism

Women with hypothyroidism are at higher risk for bilateral breast pain. Hypothyroidism is a deficiency of thyroid activity, including low levels of thyroxine. Although the exact mechanism of action on breast tissue is not understood, the breast has an affinity for the thyroid hormone and iodine. The terminal part of the duct, the acini (fluid producing cells) and the ducts are lined with cells that have iodine in them. When these levels are low, the breast becomes more sensitive to estrogen stimulation.

Some women experiencing bilateral breast pain that does not go away completely after a menstrual period or have severe breast pain may have an underlying low thyroid condition.

Diagnosing Hypothyroidism

When a woman has been unable to obtain pain relief with NSAIDS and other interventions, thyroid levels should be checked. If diagnostic tests show a deficiency, thyroid medication will be prescribed that usually relieves or greatly reduces the pain.

Symptoms associated with low thyroid function that may offer additional clues are:

- Weight gain and difficulty losing weight even with diet and exercise

- Depression, mood swings, forgetfulness

- Fatigue or exhaustion

- Chronic constipation

- Cold intolerance (feel cold when others feel warm)
- Dry, scaly skin
- Lack of perspiration during heavy exercise or hot weather
- Hair thinning
- Low sex drive
- Irregular menstrual periods or infertility

If you are experiencing a combination of these symptoms with bilateral breast pain, you should ask your healthcare provider to check for low thyroid levels. If your levels are low, supplementation with a thyroid medication brings pain relief to most women in several months.

Basal Body Temperature as a Diagnostic Tool

Some natural health practitioners have a woman take her basal body temperature for preliminary evaluation of a low thyroid condition. Broda Barnes, M.D. made this method popular years ago and it is still used as a supplementary tool to blood studies. Some endocrinologists use this evaluation when blood levels do not show a great deficiency but a combination of symptoms of low thyroid levels are present. A low basal body temperature does not prove but does suggest that the thyroid hormones may be the cause.

Instructions for taking basal body temperature:

1. Menstruating women need to begin taking their temperature on the second day of their menstrual period to be assured of accuracy since temperature rises during the period of ovulation. Menopausal women can begin at any time.

2. Place a digital or mercury thermometer beside your bed. If using a mercury thermometer, shake it down to $96°$ F or less.

3. When awakening in the morning, before you get out of bed or have anything to eat or drink, place the thermometer deep into your armpit. Leave it in place for five minutes.

4. Record your temperature on a calendar. The normal underarm temperature is $97.8°$ F - $98.2°$ F. If your temperature falls below $97.4°$ F for four days in a row, this may indicate low thyroid function.

Iodine Supplement

Since iodine is one of the main components needed for thyroid function, Dr. Tori Hudson also recommends supplementation with iodine for women with fibrocystic symptoms including pain. After reviewing the research of iodine supplements, Dr. Hudson states "aqueous iodine (3 - 6 mg daily, available by prescription only) achieved symptom relief in 74 percent of women without adverse affects on the thyroid gland." (*Women's Encyclopedia of Natural Medicine* page 93.)

Galactorrhea

Galactorrhea is a persistent milky breast discharge not related to pregnancy or lactation. The discharge comes from both breasts and through multiple openings on the nipples. The breasts become engorged with breast milk and are tender and painful. The discharge does not contain blood or pus but under a microscope it reveals fat droplets consistent with breast milk. With galactorrhea, the discharge is not just a couple of drops, but is excessive.

Prolactin is the pituitary hormone responsible for milk production. Many drugs can cause an overproduction of prolactin that in turn causes excessive milk production. Prolactin levels can increase as a result of hypothyroidism, shingles, trauma, stimulation to the breasts during sexual foreplay, or a tumor in the area of the pituitary gland.

For any woman not pregnant or recently nursing, discharge from both breasts in excessive amounts is not normal. A blood test for an evaluation of the prolactin levels will reveal the most probable cause. If the prolactin level is less than 100 ng/ml, it may be caused by medications such as Reglan (see chapter 5); medication changes may correct the problem. If the low level is caused by hypothyroidism, thyroid replacement will correct the problem.

If the level is very high, a scan of the head (MRI) is indicated to rule out a pituitary tumor. A medication, Bromocriptine (discussed earlier), is usually the first line of treatment if the discharge is promoted by a tumor. If Bromocriptine does not control or reduce the tumor and the discharge, surgery may be required.

Breast Pain Caused by Cancer

As noted earlier, breast pain associated with cancer is not common. Most cancer patients do not report pain as a common symptom, but it can occur. For this reason, all pain should always be evaluated and cancer ruled out as a possible cause.

The pain caused by cancer varies according to how large the tumor is and if it is pressing on a nerve. A tumor not visible on mammography and soft to the touch can still cause pain if it is pressing on a nerve.

Factors Increasing Risk for Breast Cancer

- Occurs in one breast only
- Lump in same breast
- Nipple discharge from same breast
- Discharge that is clear like water or has blood in it (pink to dark reddish)
- Changes in texture of skin of same breast (looks like an orange peel)
- Changes in color of skin of same breast
- Dimpling or bulging in the same breast or area of a lump
- Nipple retraction in same breast
- Increase in number or size of veins on breast skin compared to other breast
- Temperature elevation in same breast (inflammatory breast cancer)
- Excessive itching in same breast (inflammatory breast cancer)
- Increase in size of breast in short period of time (inflammatory breast cancer)
- Excessive itching of nipple (Paget's disease)
- Chronic irritation of one nipple (Paget's disease)
- Postmenopausal woman with pain in one breast
- Woman with family or personal history of breast cancer with pain in one breast not associated with menstrual cycle hormonal changes

The more of these characteristics or symptoms present, the more likely the probability that the pain may be related to a malignancy. To rule out cancer, you need a clinical exam by a trained healthcare provider, followed by a mammogram and possibly an ultrasound. Any abnormal area identified should be evaluated by a tissue biopsy to come to a definitive diagnosis. Any fine needle aspiration biopsy (FNA) or core biopsy that is negative with a mammogram that looks suspicious or a clinical exam that feels suspicious should be followed by a surgical removal of the abnormal tissue. Remember, no healthcare practitioner can diagnose disease with his or her fingers alone and there should always be agreement between the clinical exam, mammogram and/or ultrasound and biopsy results. If the three don't agree, a surgical biopsy is indicated.

Remember:

- Noncyclic pain does not correspond with changes in the menstrual cycle

- Pain may be caused by a variety of benign diseases or conditions, musculoskeletal disease or injury and medications, and physiological conditions

- Noncyclic pain usually occurs in one place in one breast; you can often put your fingers on the place that is painful

- Physiological conditions, like hypothyroidism or galactorrhea can cause pain in both breasts

- Pain with cancer is rare, but all pain should be evaluated to rule out the possibility

- Pain evaluation should consist of a thorough history, clinical breast exam and followed by a mammogram and/or ultrasound if needed and a biopsy of any abnormality for a definitive diagnosis

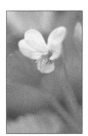

CHAPTER 4

THE CAFFEINE CONNECTION

After you have consulted with a healthcare provider and disease has been ruled out, a caffeine-free diet may reduce cyclic pain (fibrocystic changes). As previously discussed in Chapter 2, some studies have shown caffeine reduction or elimination reduces breast pain and others have not. What is important is how you respond. Some women have found that their breasts are very sensitive to caffeine products and that a diet lower in caffeine significantly reduces the amount of breast discomfort they experience. The good news about caffeine reduction is that it only requires self-discipline and does not cost anything. If you do not respond in several months you will know that this was not the cause of your cyclic bilateral pain. If your healthcare provider recommends caffeine reduction, the following information will help you understand how to best manage your diet.

- After you go on a caffeine-free diet, it will take approximately two months to show an improvement in the discomfort and pain associated with fibrocystic changes. Some women respond more slowly and may not see a change for up to a year. Others find no relief from reduced caffeine. You simply find out by trying.

- Reducing caffeine in your diet may cause you to experience headaches. It helps to gradually reduce your intake. For example, if you drink four cups of coffee a day, reduce the amount to three cups the first several days and then to two cups. Gradual reduction will minimize headaches. If you decide to eliminate caffeine completely, you may have headaches for up to seven days. This is a normal side effect from sudden and complete caffeine withdrawal.

Most people associate caffeine with coffee consumption. However, there are many products that contain high amounts of caffeine. Many women consume more caffeine from soft drinks or medications than those that drink coffee. Intake of these products also needs to be reduced or eliminated. Read carefully the labels of products to check for caffeine amounts.

Caffeine Containing Products

Product	Caffeine Milligrams
Coffee:	
Drip (5 oz.)	146
Percolated (5 oz.)	110
Instant, regular (5 oz.)	53
Decaffeinated brewed (5 oz.)	3
Decaffeinated instant (5 oz.)	2
Tea:	
Brewed (5 oz.)	60-75
Instant (5 oz.)	30
Iced tea, canned (12 oz.)	22-36
Cocoa & Chocolate:	
Cocoa (water mix) (6 oz.)	10
Chocolate bar (2-3 oz.)	10
Baking Chocolate (1 oz.)	6
Soft Drinks (12 oz.):	
Mountain Dew	52
Mello Yellow	52
Tab	52
Coke Classic	46
Diet Coke	46
Sunkist Orange	42
Shasta Cola	42
Diet Mr. Pibb	40
Mr. Pibb	40
Dr. Pepper	38
Diet Dr. Pepper	37
Pepsi Cola	37

Product	Caffeine Milligrams
Soft Drinks (12 oz.):	
Royal Crown Cola	36
Diet-Rite Cola	34
Diet Pepsi	34
Diet Mello Yellow	12
7-Up	0
Sierra Mist	0
Sprite	0
Minute Maid Orange	0
Diet 7-Up	0
Diet Sunkist Orange	0
Diet Sierra Mist	0
Fanta Orange	0
Fresca	0
Hires Root Beer	0

Non-Prescription Drugs	Caffeine Milligrams
Stimulants-standard dose:	
No-Doz	200
Vivarin	200
Pain Relievers-standard dose:	
Excedrin (2 tablets)	130
Anacin (2 tablets)	64
Midol (2 tablets)	65
Goody's Powder (1 powder)	32
BC Powder (1 powder)	32
Plain aspirin (any brand)	0
Cold Remedies:	
Dristan	32
Coryban-D	30

Herbal Products Similar to Caffeine

Some herbal supplements have been identified as having a substance identical to caffeine, guaranine. Guarana (contains 4% guaranine) and Kola Nut (cola nitida) have the same effect on the body as caffeine.

Manufacturers of these supplements have found that they can use this caffeine-like drug and market it as 'natural' or 'herbal' and never inform the consumer that it is basically chemically identical to caffeine and that the body responds to it as caffeine. This makes it much easier to market and easier to ask higher prices for the same biological effect because people do not investigate the energy enhancing properties of these herbal compounds. As with caffeine, these herbs may cause breast pain in some women. They are most often found in products marketed as energy enhancing or weight reducing products. Recognizing these names on the label may help you identify supplements that could trigger a similar caffeine reaction and be a promoting factor of your breast pain.

Remember:

■ Read the labels of all products for their caffeine contents.

■ Manufacturers of soft drinks do not have to list their amounts of caffeine.

■ Herbal products such as Guarana and Kola Nut are a type of caffeine and can have the same effects on your breasts.

■ Caffeine reduction has helped some women with breast tenderness and pain. However, it may take several months or longer to evaluate the effectiveness.

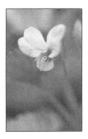

CHAPTER 5

THE DRUG CONNECTION

Investigation into the possibility of medication induced pain is one of the most under-utilized evaluations for breast pain. Healthcare providers and women concentrate on the breast as the source when promoting factors of medications and dietary products have a high incidence of being the cause of the pain.

The main categories of drugs that may cause breast changes are hormonal, blood pressure, heart, pain relievers, antibiotics, antidepressants, and gastrointestinal medications. All may cause breast tenderness and pain in some women.

Medications may be linked to cyclic or noncyclic pain. If you are taking any medication, (prescription or nonprescription) check the following lists of medications that can cause breast pain to see if your medication is listed. When you review the lists, you may find that you are taking more than one drug that can cause breast changes, increasing your potential for breast pain. If you are experiencing pain in your breasts and are presently taking any of the listed medications, you may want to discuss this with your healthcare provider. Do not stop taking any prescribed medication without consulting your healthcare provider.

However, you may decide to stop taking over-the-counter medications to evaluate your breasts' response. Most physicians recommend four to six weeks discontinuation of a medication to determine if it is the cause.

Over-The-Counter Herbal Products and Breast Pain

There has been an increase in reports of breast pain from many of the supplements used to promote weight loss (often called "fat burners") and increase energy. The Food and Drug Administration (FDA) finds that these products contain ingredients that stimulate the body in the same manner as caffeine.

Ma Huang (Ephedra Sinica or Chinese Ephedra) is a botanical source of ephedrine, pseudoephedrine, and norpseudoephedrine that is found in many herbal weight-loss products. Guarana or Kola Nut, found in many supplements, is actually a type of caffeine.

Many herbal products (especially Ginseng and Dong Quai) recommended to treat premenstrual syndrome (PMS) and menopausal symptoms may cause some women to experience an onset of breast pain. Some vitamin products marketed as "antioxidant formulas" may also contain herbs that can cause breast pain.

A diet high in soybean products or tofu may also cause some women to have breast tenderness or pain. These products produce an estrogen-like effect on the body. Some women on liquid diet products that contain a soy-protein base experience breast changes.

As with any medication, people respond differently, and some women may be very sensitive to these products. Just because a label terms a product "natural) does not mean that there will be no side effects from the product. There has been little extensive study of the numerous herbs on the market and their potential side effects. Some products may not yet be identified as causing breast changes. When evaluating the cause of your breast pain, consider the use of any medications or supplements in these categories as being possible promoters.

Identifying Drugs that
May Cause Breast Pain or Tenderness

The *PDR®* (Physician's Desk Reference) *Guide to Drug Interactions, Side Effects, Indications™* lists the drugs that may affect the breasts. Pharmaceutical manufacturers supply Medical Economics, the publisher, the information provided in the *PDR®*. Companies describe known side effects of their medications using different terminology for what may be the same breast changes.

To be precise in reporting, the *PDR®* and this book have used the manufacturers' specific wording in reporting possible side effects of their medications (* denotes a manufacturer's term) for the subcategories. All the drugs listed may cause or exacerbate breast changes and are listed by their trade names under major categories of change. Because any drug that can cause a change in the breast may result in some type of pain, we have listed all categories.

General Breast Changes

Unspecified* Breast Changes
Brevicon
Demulen
Desogen Tablets
Emcyt Capsules (10-66%)
Loestrin
Lo/Ovral Tablets
Lo/Ovral-28 Tablets
Lupron Depot-PED (Less than 2%)
Micronor Tablets
Modicon
Nordette-21 Tablets
Nordette-28 Tablets
Norinyl
Nor-Q-D Tablets
Ortho-Cept Tablets
Ortho-Cyclen Tablets
Ortho-Novum
Ortho-Tri-Cyclen
Ovral Tablets
Ovral-28 Tablets
Ovrette Tablets
Proglycem
Rogaine Topical Solution
Tri-Norinyl
Triphasil-21 Tablets
Triphasil-28 Tablets

Breast Size Changes

Unspecified*
Depo-Provera Contraceptive Injection (fewer than 1%)

Breast Atrophy*
Paxil Tablets (Rare)
Zoladex (33%)

Breast Size Reduction*
Danocrine Capsules
Supprelin Injection (2-3%)
Synarel Nasal Solution (10%)

Breast Engorgement*
Adalat CC (Less than l%)
Anafranil Capsules (Rare)
Betaseron for SC Injection
Desyrel and Desyrel Dividose
Effexor (Rare)
Haldol Decanoate
Haldol Injection, Tablets and Concentrate
Mellaril
Permax Tablets (Rare)
Ser-Ap-Es Tablets
Synarel Nasal Solution (Less than 1%)
Zoladex (Greater than 1% but less than 5%)

Enlargement*
Adapin Capsules
Aldoclor Tablets
Aldomet Ester HCI Injection
Aldomet Oral
Aldoril Tablets
Anafranil Capsules (Up to 2%)
Asendin Tablets (Less than 1%)
Brevicon
Claritin (2% or fewer)
Demser Capsules (Infrequent)
Demulen
Depakene
Depakote
Desogen Tablets
Desyrel and Desyrel Dividose
Diethylstilbestrol Tablets
Effexor (Rare)
Elavil
Emcyt Capsules (60%)
Endep Tablets

Estrace Cream and Tablets
Estraderm Transdermal System
Estradurin
Estratab Tablets
Estratest
Etrafon
Flexeril Tablets (Rare)
Indocin Capsules (Less than 1%)
Indocin I.V. (Less than 1%)
Indocin (Less than 1%)
Levlen/Tri-Levlen
Limbitrol
Loestrin
Ludiomil Tablets (Isolated reports)
Menest Tablets
Micronor Tablets
Modicon
Navane Capsules and Concentrate
Navane Intramuscular
Norinyl
Norpramin Tablets
Nor-Q D Tablets
Ogen Tablets
Ogen Vaginal Cream
Ortho-Cept Tablets
Ortho-Cyclen Tablets
Ortho Dienestrol Cream
Ortho-Est
Ortho-Novum
Ortho-Tri-Cyclen Tablets
Ovcon
PMB 200 and PMB 400
Pamelor
Premarin Intravenous
Premarin with Methyltestosterone
Premarin Tablets
Premarin Vaginal Cream
Proscar Tablets
ProSom Tablets (Rare)
Prozac Pulvules & Liquid, Oral Solution (Rare)

Sinequan
Stilphostrol Tablets and Ampules
Supprelin Injection (1-10%)
Surmontil Capsules
Synarel Nasal Solution for Central Precocious Puberty
Thorazine
Thyrel TRH (a small number)
Tofranil Ampules
Tofranil Tablets
Tofranil-PM Capsules
Triavil Tablets
Trilafon
Tri-Norinyl
Triphasil-21 Tablets
Triphasil-28 Tablets
Vivactil Tablets
Zoladex (18%)
Zoloft Tablets (Rare)

Gynecomastia* (Enlargement)

Adalat Capsules (Less than 0.5%)
Adalat C.C. (Rare)
Adapin Capsules
Aldactazide (Not infrequent)
Aldactone (Not infrequent)
Aldoclor
Aldomet Ester HCI Injection
Aldomet Oral
Aldoril Tablets
Anadrol-50 Tablets
Anafranil Capsules (Rare)
Android (Among most common)
Asendin Tablets
Atromid-S Capsules
Axid Puivules (Rare)
Betaseron for SC Injection
Calan SR Caplets (1% or less)
Calan Tablets (1% or less)
Capoten
Capozide

Catapres Tablets (About 1 in 1000)
Catapres -TTS (Less frequent)
Cipro I.V. (1% or less)
Cipro I.V. Pharmacy Bulk Package
Clinoril Tablets (Rare)
Combipres Tablets (About 1 in 1000)
Compazine
Elavil
Endep Tablets
Etrafon
Eulexin Capsules
Flexeril Tablets (Rare)
Foscavir Injection (1-5%)
Haldol Decanoate
Haldol Injection, Tablets and Concentrate
Halotestin Tablets
IBU (Ibuprofen Tablets, USP)
Indocin Capsules (Less than 1%)
Indocin I.V. (Less than 1%)
INH Tablets
Intron A (Less than 5%)
Isoptin Oral Tablets
Isoptin SR Sustained Release Tablets (1% or less)
Lanoxicaps (Occasional)
Lanoxin Elixir Pediatric
Lanoxin Injection (Occasional)
Lanoxin Injection Pediatric
Lanoxin Tablets (Occasional)
Lescol Capsules
Limbitrol
Loxitane (Rare)
Ludiomil Tablets (Isolated Reports)
Lupron Depot 3.75 mg (Among most frequent)
Lupron Depot 7.5 mg (Less than 5%)
Lupron Depot- PED (Less than 2%)
Lupron Injection (5% or more)
Matulane Capsules
Megace Oral Suspension (1-3%)
Mellaril
Mevacor Tablets (0.5-1%)

Midamor
Moban Tablets and Concentrate
Moduretic
Motrin Tablets
Myerlan Tablets
Navane Capsules and Concentrate
Navane Intramuscular
Nizoral Tablets (Less than 1%)
Norpace
Norpramin
Nydrazid Injection
Oreton Methyl (Among most common)
Orudis Capsules (Rare)
Pamelor
Pepcid Injection (Rare)
Pepcid (Rare)
Pergonal (menotropins for injection, USP)
Pravachol
Pregnyl
Prilosec Delayed-Release Capsules (Less than 1%)
Profasi (chorionic gonadotropin for injection)
Prolixin
Reglan
Rifamate
Sandimmune (1-4%)
Ser-Ap-Es Tablets
Serentil
Sinequan
Sporanox Capsules (Less than 1%)
Stelazine
Surmontil Capsules
Tagamet
Taractan
Temaril Tablets, Syrup and Spanule (extended-release)
Testoderm Testosterone (Five in 104 patients)
Testred Capsules
Thorazine
Tofranil Ampules
Tofranil-PM Capsules

Tofranil Tablets
Torecan
Trecator-SC Tablets
Triavil Tablets
Trilafon
Vaseretic Tablets
Vasotec I.V.
Vasotec Tablets (0.5%-1%)
Verelan Capsules (Less than 1%)
Vivactil Tablets
Wellbutrin Tablets (Infrequent)
Winstrol Tablets
Wytensin Tablets
Xanax Tablets
Zantac (Occasional)
Zantac Injection and Zantac Injection Premixed
Zocor Tablets
Zoloft Tablets (Rare)
Zyloprim Tablet (Less than 1%)

Breast Lumpiness

Breast Fibroadenosis*
   Ambien Tablets (Rare)
   Anafranil Capsules (Rare)
   Kerlone Tablets (Less than 2%)
Fibrocystic Breasts*
   Betaseron for SC Injection (3%)
   Levlen/Tri-Levlen
   Micronor Tablets
   Modicon
   Ortho-Cyclen Tablets
   Ortho-Novum
   Ortho-Tri-Cyclen Tablets
   Permax Tablets (Infrequent)
   Prozac Pulvules, Liquid, Oral Solution (Infrequent)
Breast Lumps*
   Depo/Provera Contraceptive Injection
   Levlen/Tri-Levlen

Ortho-Cyclen Tablets
Ortho-Est
Ortho-Cyclen Tablets

Breast Pain or Tenderness

Breast Pain*

Anafranil (Up to 1%)
Betaseron for SC Injection (7%)
Cardura Tablets (Less than 0.5%)
Clozaril Tablets (Less than 1%)
Cognex Capsules (Infrequent)
Imdur (Less than or equal to 5%)
Lupron Depot 7.5 mg.
Paxil Tablets
Pentasa (Less than 1%)
Procardia XL Extended Release Tablets (Less than 1%)
Prozac Pulvules and Liquid, Oral Solution (Infrequent)
Sporanox Capsules (Less than 1%)
Zoladex (7%)
Zoloft Tablets (Rare)

Breast Tenderness*

Amen Tablets (Rare)
Azactam for Injection (Less than 1%)
Brevicon
Bumex (0.1%)
Cycrin Tablets (Rare)
Demulen (Among most common)
Depo-Provera Contraceptive Injection
Desogen Tablets
Diethylstilbestrol Tablets
Emcyt Capsules (66%)
Estrace Cream and Tablets
Estrace Vaginal Cream
Estraderm Transdermal System
Estratab Tablets
Estratest
Indocin (Less than 1%)
Indocin Capsules

Indocin I.V.
Levlen/Tri-Levlen
Lo/Ovral Tablets
Lo/Ovral-28 Tablets
Loniten Tablets (Less than 1%)
Lupron Depot 7.5 mg.
Lupron Injection (5% or more)
Menest Tablets
Metrodin
Micronor Tablets
Modicon
Norinyl
Norlutate
Nor-Q D Tablets
Ogen Tablets
Ogen Vaginal Cream
Ortho-Cept Tablets
Ortho-Cyclen Tablets
Ortho Dienestrol Cream
Ortho-Est.
Ortho-Novum
Ortho-Tri-Cyclen Tablets
Ovcon Ovral Tablets
Ovral-28 Tablets
Ovrette Tablets
PMB 200 and PMB 400
Premarin Intravenous
Premarin Vaginal Cream
Premarin with Methyltestosterone
Premarin Tablets
Prostin E2 Suppository
Provera Tablets (Rare)
Serophene (clomiphene citrate tablets)
Stilphostrol Tablets and Ampules
Testoderm Testosterone Transdermal System
Levlen/Tri-Levlen
Tri-Norinyl
Triphasil-21 Tablets
Triphasil-28 Tablets
Zoladex (Greater than 1% but less than 5%)

Breast Discharge

Breast Secretions*
Brevicon
Danocrine Capsules (Rare)
Demulen
Desogen Tablets
Diethylstilbestrol Tablets
Dienestrol Cream
Estratest
Levlen/Tri-Levlen
Loestrin
Menest Tablets
Micronor Tablets
Modicon
Norinyl
Norplant System
Nor-Q D Tablets
Ogen Vaginal Cream
Ortho-Cept Tablets
Ortho-Cyclen
Ortho Dienestrol Cream
Ortho-Est 0.625 Tablets
Ortho-Est 1.25 Tablets
Ortho-Novum
Ortho-Tri-Cyclen Tablets
Ovcon
PMB 200 and PMB 400
Premarin Intravenous
Premarin Vaginal Cream
Premarin with Methyltestosterone
Stilphostrol Tablets and Ampules
Supprelin Injection
Tri-Norinyl

Bleeding from the Nipple*
Ceclor Pulvules & Suspension
Depo-Provera Contraceptive Injection (Less than 1%)

Galactorrhea*

Adapin Capsules
Amen Tablets (Rare)
Asendin Tablets (Less than 1%)
BuSpar (Rare)
Calan SR Caplets (1% or less)
Calan Tablets (1% or less)
Compazine
Cycrin Tablets (Rare)
Demser Capsules (Infrequent)
Depakene Capsules & Syrup
Depakote
Depo-Provera Contraceptive Injection (Fewer than 1%)
Depo-Provera Sterile Aqueous Suspension
Elavil
Endep Tablets
Etrafon
Flexeril Tablets (Rare)
Haldol Decanoate
Haldol Injection, Tablets and Concentrate
Isoptin SR Sustained Release Tablets (1% or less)
Limbitrol
Loxitane (Rare)
Ludiomil Tablets (Isolated reports)
Mellaril
Moban Tablets and Concentrate
Norpramin Tablets
Pamelor
Proglycem
Prolixin Oral Concentrate
Provera Tablets (Rare)
Reglan
Sandostatin Injection (Less than 1%)
Seldane Tablets
Seldane D Extended-ReleaseTablets
Serentil
Sinequan
Stelazine
Surmontil

Tofranil Ampules
Tofranil PM Capsules
Tofranil Tablets
Triavil Tablets
Trilafon
Vivactil Tablets
Xanax Tablets

Drug information: Reprinted with permission. Copyright *PDR® Guide to Drug Interactions, Side Effects, Indications*™ 1995 edition, published by Medical Economics, Montvale, New Jersey 07646. All rights reserved.

Remember:

■ Women respond differently to medications. Some women will respond with changes in their breasts while others will not.

■ Most medication-induced breast changes will occur in both breasts. However, one breast may have more exaggerated symptoms.

■ Understanding medications and the potential changes they may cause in your breasts could save you much anxiety and thousands of dollars in medical costs by avoiding having the problem evaluated with expensive diagnostic tests.

■ Learning the cause of the change in your breasts will often make the symptoms much more bearable.

■ Stopping some medications may bring relief in days. However, it may take four to six weeks after stopping other medications to evaluate the effect they may have on your breast problem. Times vary because of different medications and different women's responses to them.

■ Do not stop any prescription medication without consulting your healthcare provider.

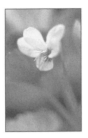

CHAPTER 6

IDENTIFYING YOUR PAIN

As you can see, there are many causes of breast pain. For some women it will be easy to identify the cause. For others, it may take a period of observing one's lifestyle and several diagnostic tests to find the cause.

Remember, the majority of pain is not related to cancer but to benign causes; but all persistent pain needs evaluation. Often, knowing the cause will make the pain bearable. Not knowing is what seems unbearable. You can help your healthcare provider determine which type of pain you are experiencing by having your history ready. When you go to see your healthcare provider, be prepared by bringing as much information as possible to help them.

Start by giving a complete breast health and breast pain history:

- Present age and menopausal status

- Date of last menstrual period or estimated due date of next period

- Birth control or hormone replacement history

- History of breastfeeding

- Family history of breast or ovarian cancer on mother and father's side for two generations

- Present prescription medications and over-the-counter products including herbal and caffeine containing products

- Any previous breast problems: lump, discharge, or previous breast biopsy (take copy of final pathology report if available)

- History of surgery for breast reduction or cancer

- History of breast implants (previously removed or presently in place)

- Date of last mammogram or ultrasound (if physician does not have report, call facility for copy before your appointment)

■ Report any abnormalities that you have felt or observed: lump, discharge, itching, dimpling, change in size, change in texture of skin, change in color, or an area of irritation that does not go away.

Pain History:

■ Provide calendar record if you have kept one.

■ Date pain first experienced and time in your cycle if you remember.

■ Is pain in the breast (unilateral) or both breasts (bilateral)?

■ Does it hurt in one spot or the whole breast?

■ Does it radiate to other areas?

■ Show your healthcare provider where it is painful by placing your finger or hand on your breast(s).

■ Was the onset sudden or gradual?

■ Is pain near the surface of the breast or deep in the breast?

■ Report any injury to the breast or back (spine) around the time of onset.

■ Is the pain sporadic or continuous?

■ What makes the pain worse? (Moving chest wall, touching area, taking a deep breath, jogging, or walking fast.)

■ What you have done to try to relieve pain.
  (Aspirin/Tylenol®/Ibuprofen, no activity, wearing bra, etc.)

■ On a scale of 1 (no pain) to 10 (severe pain), rate your pain at time of your exam and also rate the pain at the highest level you experience it.

A complete history is very helpful to a healthcare provider. This provides them the foundation for clinical evaluation. A thorough clinical breast exam is the next step of evaluation by a provider. If your mammogram is not recent and pain is unilateral it should be repeated. If the pain is bilateral, and the mammogram was recent (several months), the provider may feel that this is sufficient. If you have never had a mammogram and the provider feels that it would be helpful to rule out any thing not palpable or to evaluate an area of concern, one will be ordered. Ultrasound is another excellent tool for evaluation of an area of concern. It may be used after a mammogram, or alone in younger women and on areas the provider feels need further exploration.

Occasionally, if a healthcare provider feels that additional information is needed that can be found or clarified through a breast MRI, (Magnetic Resonance Imaging) one may be ordered. This is an imaging test that uses strong magnets to produce the images. There is no preparation for the test and no compression is used during the exam. A contrast agent (dye) may be injected into a vein before the test. You will lie still as the large magnet takes pictures. This test is ordered only after all other diagnostic tests have failed to provide any answers. An MRI does not replace mammography; it only supplements information gained from a mammogram. An MRI is a very expensive test at this time and has limitations in that it does not identify microcalcifications. It is very helpful when used in women with implants to determine if the implants are intact.

When these diagnostic methods are completed, your healthcare provider will determine if there is any evidence of breast disease, if there is a need for a biopsy, or if your pain is one from another cause. This is where the search begins for all of the different promoting causes we have discussed in this book. If you have not kept a calendar record of your pain, activities, diet, and medications, you should do so immediately. It will be helpful in the investigation. You and your healthcare provider will become partners in solving the mystery of your breast pain. For some women this may take a day for the initial evaluation and for others several months to track down the cause. The main thing is that you can determine what is causing your breast pain and take steps to reduce or eliminate it.

If for any reason your healthcare provider fails to recognize the importance of identifying your pain, seek a second opinion. Some healthcare providers fail to take an interest in breast pain, knowing that most often it is not associated with cancer. They feel their time is best-spent detecting cancer. However, many healthcare providers are very interested and skilled in tracking down the cause of pain not caused by cancer. Call your local breast center and ask if they can make a referral to someone who specializes in detecting and diagnosing breast pain.

Types and Descriptions of Breast Pain

Cyclic Pain

(usually both breasts, may be greater in one breast)

Fibrocystic	Heavy, full of milk, dull, aching, tender. May also be felt from underarm to elbow.

Noncyclic Pain

(usually one breast)

Pinched Back Nerve (Back Injury)	Sharp, radiating pain from shoulder into upper or lower breast.
Costochondritis	Tender, aching, sometimes sharp pain near breastbone. Increases when breathing deeply or lifting hands above head.
Breast Injury	Sore, bruised or stabbing pain. Breast may turn bluish/red and then goldish/yellow in area of injury.
Mastitis (infection)	Throbbing, redness and warmth of tissues. May be generalized or in one quadrant. Fever and flu-like symptoms.
Abscess (infection)	Throbbing, shooting pain, redness and warmth of tissues. Fever and flu-like symptoms.
Duct Ectasia	Itching, burning, drawing pain with thick cream/green/gray/brownish discharge. One or both breasts. One or all ducts on nipple. Late stage nipple inversion.
Mondor's Syndrome	Throbbing with sharp pains with raised rope-like cord through breast caused by inflammation in a vein from a blood clot.

Comparison of Cyclic, Noncyclic and Musculoskeletal Pain

FEATURE	CYCLIC	NONCYCLIC	MUSCULOSKELETAL
Age of Onset	20s-30s	30s-40s	Any Age
Location	Bilateral Upper Outer Area	Unilateral One Area	Usually Unilateral Often Near Breastbone
Area of Breast	Spread Out	One Spot	Different Parts of Breast
Type of Pain	Dull, Aching	Sharp, Stabbing	Burning, Aching
Status	Premenopausal	Pre- or Post-Menopausal	Any Age
Hormone Treatment	Responds Well	Minimal Response	No Response
Ibuprofen or Aspirin	Some Help	Some Help	Very Helpful

Breast Pain Treatments

The following drugs/vitamins have been used with varying results in the treatment of breast pain in different clinical trials. Dosages are those reported in the literature that were used in studies. **These are not recommendations from EduCare.** Some require lab values to monitor patient. Check with your healthcare provider before using any medication.

DRUG	TYPE	ACTION	DOSE
Vitamin E	Alpha Tocopherol Vitamin E	Slow onset, continuous treatment	600 IU per day
Vitamin B1 and 6 or B Complex	Vitamins	Slow onset, continuous treatment	100 mg daily
Vitamin A	Vitamin	Slow onset	50,000 IU per day 2 months
Evening Primrose Oil* (Gamma-Linolenic Acid)	Essential fatty acid	Slow onset, continuous treatment	3 grams per day
Iodine (Molecular)	Mineral		0.07 - 0.09 mg/kg per day

Testosterone	Male Hormone	Short term use	40 mg twice daily Testosterone Cream
Danazol	Male Hormone	Blocks female hormones	200 mg per day
Levothyroxine	Thyroid replacement	Balances thyroid hormones	0.01 per day for 2 months
Ibuprofen	Anti-inflammatory	Days to week	400 mg every 4-6 hours
Tamoxifen	Anti-Estrogen	Blocks estrogen	20 mg per day
Progesterone (oral) Progesterone Cream	Hormone	Balances estrogen in ratio to progesterone	20 mg per day orally 10 days before period. Cream rubbed into breasts or inner thighs 10 days prior to period

* Most preferred treatment

Benign Conditions Causing Breast Pain

CONDITION	DESCRIPTION	SYMPTOM	DIAGNOSTIC METHOD	TREATMENT
Cysts	Fluid-filled sac	Feels like a soft to firm lump that moves freely; may be painless or painful	• Clinical exam • Mammogram • Ultrasound	• If small, none • If large, fine needle aspiration
Fibroadenoma	Firm lump	Feels very firm and moves freely; usually painless unless pressing on a nerve	• Clinical exam • Mammogram • Ultrasound	• Biopsy required for definite diagnosis (core) • May or may not be surgically removed
Mastitis	Infection of the milk glands	• Pink to red skin, tenderness, and pain starting in one quadrant of the breast • Fever and flu-like symptoms	• Breastfeeding or recent history of nursing	• Antibiotics immediately • Wear bra day & night
Galactocele	Firm milk-filled sac	Palpable lump, moves freely	• Breastfeeding or recent history of nursing	• None, if small and resolves • Fine needle aspiration if large and does not resolve

Duct Ectasia	Inflammation of milk ducts (may range from one orifice on one breast to multiple orifices on both breasts	• Discharge ranging from gray or green to dark brownish • Pain under areola • Thick and sticky discharge • Itching nipple • Redness in area of discharge during acute stage • Late stage: nipple retraction, abscess, or breast fistula	• Symptoms • Mammogram • Ultrasound • Culture	• Antibiotics • Bra to stabilize breast
Breast Abscess	Collection of pus in one area from infection	• Pink to red skin, tenderness and pain starting in one quadrant of breast • Fever, flu-like symptoms • Lump in area of pain	• Symptoms • Culture	• Antibiotics immediately • Wear bra day & night
Mondor's Disease	Inflammation of a breast vein (most common thoracoepigastric)	• Pain, often severe and in path of vein • Palpable, round cord-like, traversing breast • Tenderness over cord area • Skin retraction along path of cord	• Symptoms • Mammogram if tolerated • Ultrasound	• Pain medications • Wear bra day & night • Restricting activities and arm movements on affected side

Conditions Mistaken for Breast Pain

CONDITION	DESCRIPTION	SYMPTOM	DIAGNOSTIC METHOD	TREATMENT
Costochondritis	Inflammation of cartilage between ribs near sternum	• Pain in chest area • Pain increases with movement of rib cage or deep breath • Pressure on sternum produces pain	• Symptoms • Physical exam • Chest x-ray • EKG possible to rule out heart problems	• Pain medications (non-steroidal anti-inflammatory drugs) • Wear bra day & night • Restriction of movement of arms and rib cage • Steroid injections occasionally
Pinched Nerve Back	Pain in breast and/or arm	Noncyclic pain; may be sharp or nagging in breast	• Cervical spine exam • X-ray or MRI of back • Breast disease ruled out	Treatment of underlying problem
Breast Injury	Direct blow to breast	• Pain • Bruise • Lump, if hematoma (collection of blood)	• History of trauma • Physical Exam • Ultrasound	• Pain medication • Possible aspiration of hematoma if painful

Back Injury	Injury to back or spine	Pain (sharp or nagging in breast and/or arm)	• History of trauma • Physical Exam • Breast disease ruled out • X-rays or MRI of back	Treatment of underlying problem
Scoliosis, Osteoporosis	Pain referred from back	Pain, sharp or nagging in breast and arm	• History of diagnosis of scoliosis or osteoporosis • Breast disease ruled out	Treatment of underlying disease process
Heart Problems	• Pain (angina) • Congestive heart failure	• Pain in chest area • Chronic sensation of fullness in chest area	• Symptoms • Clinical Exams • EKG • Breast disease ruled out	Treatment of underlying disease process
Gastrointestinal Hiatal hernia, Reflux condition, Ulcer	Pain in chest area	Pressure pain or burning pain	• Symptoms • Physical Exam • Breast disease ruled out • X-rays of esophagus and stomach • Esophagogastroscopy (tube with viewing light inserted, biopsy capability)	Treatment of underlying disease process

Conditions Mistaken for Breast Pain

CONDITION	DESCRIPTION	SYMPTOM	DIAGNOSTIC METHOD	TREATMENT
Post-Surgical Pain Biopsy Site Lumpectomy Reduction Augmentation	Sharp or dull pain in post-surgical breast	• Sharp and shooting, burning, or dull aching pain • Occasional or chronic	• History of surgery • Physical exam • Mammogram • Ultrasound	• Non-steroidal anti-inflammatory medications • Lidocaine/steroid injections for persistent pain
Breast Implants	Chest wall irritation from implants	Chronic unilateral or bilateral pain	• Symptoms • History • Breast disease ruled out • MRI	• Non-steroidal anti-inflammatory medications • Removal of implants if chronic
Herpes Zoster (Shingles) Breast or unilateral chest wall	• Sudden onset of sharp pain with burning sensation in one breast • History of chickenpox	• Chills and fever • Broad streak of reddened skin in nerve path (unilateral) • 4-5 days after onset, painful, itching blisters appear	• Symptoms • History • Breast disease ruled out	• Pain medications • Viral medications • Cortisone medications • Topical medications for itching

Silicone Granulomas	Collection of free silicone leaked from implant causing an inflammatory reaction	• Silicone implants in place, or removed. • Pain in area from implant • May or may not have palpable lump • Visible on imaging	• History of silicone implant in place or removed • Mammogram • Ultrasound • MRI • Breast disease ruled out • FNA possible	May or may not be surgically removed
Implant Contracture	Fibrous shell forms around implant and causes it to change shape which may be painful	• Implants in breast • Visible or palpable changes in breast • Visible on imaging	• MRI	Surgical intervention to reduce contracture or to remove implant
Galactorrhea	Pain and tenderness with bilateral breast engorgement and discharge	Bilateral spontaneous, bilateral discharge of excessive amount of breast milk in non-pregnant or nursing women	• Prolactin levels • Medications that promote discharge • MRI if levels high for pituitary tumor	• Remove stimulation for prolactin production • Change medication if cause • Bromocriptine • Possible surgery

Remember:

- A thorough history is the first step to evaluating your breast pain; be prepared when visiting your healthcare provider with information needed

- A combination of breast exams, mammography, ultrasound, MRI, blood studies or biopsy may be necessary to arrive at a final diagnosis

- A healthcare provider needs you as a working partner to help determine the cause of your pain

- You need and deserve a healthcare provider that is dedicated to finding the cause of your breast pain

REFERENCES

Ajmera P.R., Larbi A.B., Gebhardt G., et al., *PDR Guide to Drug Interactions, Side Effects, Indications*. Montvale, NJ: Medical Economics Company, Inc. 2002.

Bennett B.B., Steinbach B.G, Hardt N.S., and Haigh L.S., *Breast Disease for Clinicians*, New York, NY: McGraw Hill, 2001

Bland K.I. and Copeland III E.M., *The Breast*. Philadelphia, PA: W. B. Saunders Company, 1991.

Bohmert H.H. and Leis Jr. P.H., *Breast Cancer*. New York, NY: Thieme Medical, 1989.

Food and Drug Administration Medwatch, FDA Medical Bulletin, *Botanical Dietary Supplement Adverse Effects*, 994. 24 (No2): 3, Drugdex (R) Editorial Staff.

Dixon J.M. and Morrow M., *Breast Disease: A Problem-Based Approach*. New York: W.B. Saunders, 1999

Spratt J.S. and Donegan W.L., *Cancer of the Breast*. Philadelphia, PA: W.B. Saunders Company, l995.

Lippman M.E., Morrow M., Hellman S., and Harris J.R., *Diseases of the Breast*. Philadelphia, PA: Lippincott-Raven, 1996.

Hudson, Tori, *Women's Encyclopedia of Natural Medicine*. Los Angeles, CA: Keats Publishing, 1999

Hughes L.E., Mansel R.E., and Webster D.J.T., *Benign Disorders and Diseases of the Breast*. Philadelphia, PA: W.B. Saunders, 2000

Hunt K.K., Robb G.L, Strom E.A., and Ueno N.T. *Breast Cancer* (M.D. Anderson Cancer Series). New York, NY: Springer-Verlag, 2001

Marchant D.J., *Contemporary Management of Breast Diseases: Benign Disease*. Philadelphia, PA: W. B. Saunders, 1994.

Physicians Desk Reference, Breast Cancer Disease Management, Montvale, NJ: Medical Economics Company, Inc. 2002

Pazdur R., Coia L.R., Hoskins W.J., and Wagman L.D., *Cancer Management: A Multidisciplinary Approach*. Melville, NY: PRR, 2002

PDR for Herbal Medicines, Montvale, NJ: Medical Economics Company, Inc. 1998

Silva O.E. and Zurrida S., *Breast Cancer: A Practical Guide*, New York, NY: Elsevier Science Ltd., 2000

GLOSSARY

It is helpful if you understand the medical terminology used in breast care. A list of the most common medical terms used in breast care follows. If you do not understand the technical language used by healthcare providers, ask them to explain what they mean. This will enable you to be a more effective partner in monitoring your breasts.

A

Areola - The darker, circular area of skin surrounding the nipple.

B

Bilateral - Having two sides or pertaining to both sides.

Biopsy - A procedure to obtain a sample of tissues to be evaluated by a pathologist for disease. Breast biopsies may be by fine needle aspiration, core biopsy, stereotactic core biopsy, incisional surgical biopsy or excisional biopsy.

> **FNA (Fine Needle Aspiration)** - Procedure that removes cells or fluid from tissues through a needle with an empty syringe. Cells or breast fluid are extracted by pulling back on plunger and are then analyzed by a physician.

> **Core Biopsy** - Removal of a piece of a lump or calcifications with a large coring needle. The core tissue samples are sent to the lab to see if they are benign or malignant.

> **Surgical Biopsy** - Biopsy may or may not be frequently performed under general anesthesia. The surgeon makes an incision above the suspicious area and manually removes the lump or questionable tissue. Also known as incisional or excisional biopsy.

Benign breast disease - A condition of the breast that is not cancer and is not life-threatening.

Breast Abscess - A collection of pus contained in one area of the breast. It will feel hard, painful, and warm to the touch. Most commonly found under the areola in the area of the ducts.

C

Cellulitis - Infection occurring in soft tissues. The surgical arm has an increased risk for cellulitis because of the removal of lymph nodes during breast cancer surgery. Pain, swelling, and warmth occur in the area.

Clinical exam - Breast exam by a healthcare provider.

Costochondral Junctions - Areas in the ribcage where the cartilage, which holds the ribs together, connects with them.

Costochondritis - Inflammation of cartilage between ribs causing pain.

Culture - An evaluation of cell samples in a lab to determine types of microorganisms present (bacteria, viruses, algae, fungi, and protozoa).

Cyclic Pain - Pain that occurs in cycles corresponding to changes in hormones during the monthly menstrual cycle.

Cyst - An abnormal, benign, sac-like structure that contains liquid or semi-solid material; Lumps in the breast are often found to be harmless cysts.

D

Duct - A narrow conduit, tubular in shape, that conveys hormonal secretions out of a gland.

Duct Ectasia - An inflammation of the ducts of the breast accompanied by nipple discharge. Other symptoms may include itching, pain, or nipple inversion.

E

EKG - Electrocardiogram of the heart detects and records electrical potential and activity of the heart during contraction. The EKG machine records and prints out a record for evaluation by a physician.

Estrogen - A female hormone secreted by the ovaries which is essential for menstruation, reproduction and the development of secondary sex characteristics, such as breasts. Some patients with breast cancer are given drugs to suppress the production of estrogen in their bodies.

Estrogen Dominance - Levels of estrogen are high in comparison to progesterone.

Estrogen Replacement Therapy - (ERT) Medication given to replace or supplement normal levels of estrogen in women.

F

Fibroadenoma - A noncancerous, solid tumor most commonly found in younger women.

Fibrocystic Changes - A noncancerous breast condition caused by female hormones causing pain, tenderness, lumpiness, or cysts. Condition fluctuates with the menstrual cycle.

G

Galactocele - A clogged milk duct forming a cyst filled with milk that occurs during lactation (breast milk production).

Galactorrhea - Breast discharge of breast milk from both breasts.

H

Healthcare Provider - A trained person who provides health care services. Physician, nurse, nurse practitioner, physicians' assistant and other specialties.

Hematoma - A collection of blood that can form in a wound after surgery, an aspiration, or from an injury.

Hormones - Chemicals secreted by various organs in the body that help regulate growth, metabolism and reproduction. Most common female hormones are estrogen, progesterone and prolactin.

Hypothyroidism - Condition of low thyroid hormones in the body causing low metabolic rate, fatigue, cold intolerance and breast pain.

I

Inflammatory Breast Cancer - A very aggressive (though rare) form of breast cancer. This cancer can cause pain, which may be accompanied by rapid changes in the texture and color of the breast. Itching and increases in breast size are also symptoms.

L

Lobule - A small lobe or subdivision of a lobe; in this text it refers to sac-like areas at the branching end of each duct which are filled with the acini, the milk-producing structures of the breast.

Lumpectomy - A surgical procedure in which only the cancerous tumor and an area of surrounding tissue is removed. Usually the surgeon will remove some of the underarm lymph nodes at the same time. This procedure is also referred to as a tylectomy.

M

MammaCare® - A modification of the traditional breast self-exam developed as a result of research funded by the National Cancer Institute. Considered to be the most thorough of the self exam methods.

Mammography - X-ray of the breasts by a special machine that produces pictures of the internal parts of the breasts.

Mastalgia/Mastodynia - Pain in the breast.

Mastectomy - Surgical removal of the entire breast and some of the surrounding tissue.

Mastitis - Infection occurring in the breast. Pain, tenderness, swelling, redness and warmth may be observed. Usually related to infection and will respond to antibiotic treatment.

Menopause - Period of life when menstrual periods stop. Average age of onset is 52 years.

Microcalcifications - Particles seen on a mammogram that looks like small white spots on the picture. Microcalcifications are from calcium deposits caused by death of breast cells; they may be benign or malignant. When they are clustered in one small area or follow the pattern of a breast duct they are checked more closely for disease in the breast.

Mondor's Syndrome - An inflamed vein in the breast, may occur after trauma, muscular strain, radiation therapy, or surgical procedures. May also be called "breast phlebitis" or "superficial periphlebitis."

Musculoskeletal - Pertaining to muscles and skeleton of the body.

Noncyclic Pain - Pain that does not occur in cycles corresponding with female menstrual cycle.

N

NSAIDs - An acronym for "**n**onsteroidal **a**nti-**i**nflammatory **d**rug". Medications under this classification include ibuprofen and aspirin.

O

Oncology - The area of medical expertise dealing with the treatment of cancer.

Ovulation - Period of time (midcycle) in female menstrual cycle when an egg is released from an ovary.

P

Premenopausal - Female who has menstrual cycles.

Palpable - Can be felt by touching.

Perimenopausal - Period several years before onset of menopause.

Prolactin - A female hormone secreted by the pituitary gland that causes the production of breast milk.

Progesterone - Female hormone produced by the ovaries during a specific time in the menstrual cycle. Causes the uterus to prepare for pregnancy and the breasts to get ready to produce milk.

Prostaglandins - Components in body that have an important role in regulating cell activities, especially in the inflammatory response that causes pain.

S

Screening Evaluations - Exams used to detect breast disease-clinical breast exam, mammogram, ultrasound, and occasionally MRI.

T

Tietze's Syndrome - Inflammation of cartilage between ribs that has pain and swelling at the rib cartilage junction.

U

Unilateral - Affecting only one side.

Ultrasound - An imaging exam that uses high-frequency sound waves to create pictures of internal organs on a screen.

INDEX

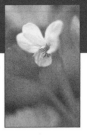

Breast Pain *Description*

Name: _____ Age: _____

Birth Control Pills: ☐ yes   ☐ no
Menopausal: ☐ yes   ☐ no
Estrogen Replacement: ☐ yes   ☐ no

Kind of Pain:

Describe your pain by checking the following descriptive terms:

- ☐   Tender to touch _____
- ☐   Dull, Aching _____
- ☐   Throbbing _____
- ☐   Burning sensation _____
- ☐   Sharp, stabbing _____
- ☐   Other _____

Where does it hurt?

Mark on this diagram the area where you feel the pain. If the pain radiates from the breast, draw an arrow in the direction it radiates.

☐ One breast

☐ Both breasts

☐ Pain localized

☐ Pain generalized

☐ Near surface of breast

☐ Pain deep in breast

How and when did the pain begin?

Sudden onset of pain	☐ yes	☐ no
Gradual increase over past few months	☐ yes	☐ no
Pain increasing	☐ yes	☐ no
Breast pain started _____		

When is it painful?

At rest	☐ yes	☐ no
Walking or exercising	☐ yes	☐ no
Taking a deep breath or stretching	☐ yes	☐ no
Only when touched or with movement	☐ yes	☐ no
Keeps you from going to sleep	☐ yes	☐ no
Awakens you from sleep	☐ yes	☐ no

What relieves the pain?

Aspirin/Tylenol®/Ibuprofen	☐ yes	☐ no
Wearing a bra	☐ yes	☐ no
No activity	☐ yes	☐ no
Heat	☐ yes	☐ no
Cold	☐ yes	☐ no
Other _____		

Do you drink or take?

Coffee	☐ yes	☐ no
Soft Drinks containing caffeine	☐ yes	☐ no
Herbal products	☐ yes	☐ no
Over-the-counter pain/diet/energy pills	☐ yes	☐ no
Supplemental estrogen/birth control pills	☐ yes	☐ no
Medications: List _____		

_____

_____

Fill in this information for your healthcare provider. This will be helpful in gathering clues, patterns and connections which can help identify the probable cause of your breast pain.

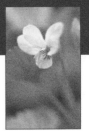

Breast Pain *Assessment Chart*

Name: _____ Age: _____

Date Started: _____ Date Completed: _____

Record your daily amount of breast pain on this chart. Careful recording of the pain will enable your healthcare provider to determine possible causes.

Mark the following information on your calendar:

■ Day you begin your menstrual period - MP1 (menstrual period day 1).

■ Day your menstrual period ends - MPS (menstrual period stopped).

■ If you are menopausal, mark MX at the beginning of the chart.

■ Chart pain on a scale, rating pain in a range from 0 (no pain) to 10 (severe pain).

■ Chart the area in the breast where the pain occurs; see breast diagram below for numbers. The breast is divided into four quadrants. You may select one or multiple areas of the breasts. Example: LB 1, 3, 4.

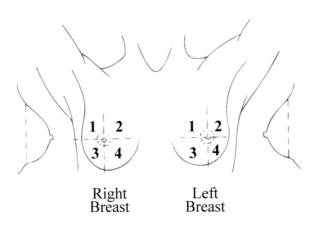

Right Breast   Left Breast

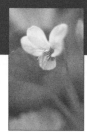

Breast Pain *Assessment Chart*

- Note time of day pain is experienced:
  AM (midnight to noon)
  PM (noon to midnight)
  AD (all day)

- On each day pain is experienced, record unusual physical activities performed.

- Note any unusual dietary changes on days pain is experienced (more or less consumption of caffeine, etc.)

- Note any medication usage (cold pills, herbal products, prescription medications. etc.).

Example of one day's charting:
Saturday, January 1
MP1 (menstrual period day 1)
Pain #6
LB3 (left breast, area 3)
AD (all day)
Tennis
1 Coffee, 2 Cokes, Herbal Tea, Cold Pills X2

Charting Abbreviations:

AD	All Day
AM	Midnight to Noon
LB	Left Breast
MP1	Menstrual Period Day 1
MPS	Menstrual Period Stopped
MX	Menopausal
PM	Noon to Midnight
RB	Right Breast

EduCare *Worksheet*

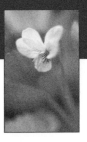

Breast Pain *Assessment Calendar*

	Week 1	Week 2
Sunday		
Monday		
Tuesday		
Wednesday		
Thursday		
Friday		
Saturday		

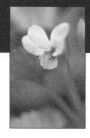

Breast Pain *Assessment Calendar*

	Week 3	Week 4
Sunday		
Monday		
Tuesday		
Wednesday		
Thursday		
Friday		
Saturday		

EduCare *Worksheet*

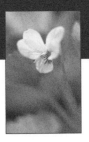

Breast Pain *Assessment Calendar*

	Week 1	Week 2
Sunday		
Monday		
Tuesday		
Wednesday		
Thursday		
Friday		
Saturday		

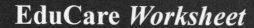

EduCare *Worksheet*

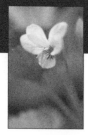

Breast Pain *Assessment Calendar*

	Week 3	Week 4
Sunday		
Monday		
Tuesday		
Wednesday		
Thursday		
Friday		
Saturday		

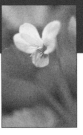

Drugs That I Take

List any medications that have been prescribed by a healthcare provider, over-the-counter medications, and herbal products that you take either occasionally or on a regular basis.

Prescription Drugs: _____

_____

_____

_____

_____

_____

_____

Over-the-Counter Drugs: _____

_____

_____

_____

_____

_____

_____

Herbal Products: _____

_____

_____

_____

_____

_____

_____

Notes